Praise for The Adaptation Diet by Charles A. Moss, MD

If you have no hope you can ever lose that weight and feel at peace, read *The Adaptation Diet* by Dr. Charles Moss. It provides clear, concise suggestions that can help you shed not only the pounds but also many of your other health concerns. Yes, you are holding the book that has proven sensible recommendations and explanations to resolve many medical challenges. Turn your life around today, by simply trying this diet.

Doris J. Rapp, MD,
Author of Our Toxic World, A Wake Up Call.

The Adaptation Diet offers a unique perspective on weight loss, pointing out the weight-gaining effects of "dietary stress", and how to deal with them. Going 'way beyond just calorie control, Dr. Charles Moss points out that dietary stress reduction—with or without calorie reduction—will result in significant and sustained weight loss.

What's dietary stress? It's food that leads to sustained increases in cortisol, the principal stress-response hormone, which is also a principal "weight gainer" hormone. And which foods do that? Unfortunately, most of what supermarkets sell—refined foods, processed foods, sugar and chemical-added foods, pro-inflammatory foods, and even "good-for-you" foods to which you're allergic, but don't know it!

The Adaptation Diet then tells us which foods and supplements actually reduce the food-stress induced over-active cortisol response, allowing that elusive goal, weight loss, to happen while at the same time improving your health. If you want to lose weight, *The Adaptation Diet* is an excellent place to start!

Jonathan Wright, MD,
Editor, "Nutrition & Healing Newsletter".

"The Adaptation Diet provides user-friendly but scientifically supported information that not only correlates so many of our modern day diseases with our stressful environment, but more importantly, gives readers the tools to undo the damage."

—David Perlmutter, MD, FACN, ABIHM
Author of The Better Brain Book

The
Adaptation
Diet

The
Adaptation
Diet

The Complete Prescription
for Reducing Stress, Feeling Great and Protecting Yourself Against Obesity, Diabetes and Heart Disease

Charles A. Moss, MD

iUniverse, Inc.
New York   Bloomington

iUniverse books may be ordered through booksellers or by contacting:

iUniverse
1663 Liberty Drive
Bloomington, IN 47403
www.iuniverse.com
1-800-Authors (1-800-288-4677)

ISBN: 978-1-4401-9231-9 (sc)
ISBN: 978-1-4401-9232-6 (ebook)

Printed in the United States of America

iUniverse rev. date: 01/26/2010

Dedicated to my mother, Helen Moss, for her unconditional love and many nutritious home-cooked meals.

About the Author

Charles A. Moss, MD, is a pioneer in the use of therapeutic nutrition in medicine. Since 1978 he has helped his patients regain health and manage their weight through dietary changes that reduce maladaptation (the long-term elevation of cortisol and other stress hormones that increases the risk for chronic disease). He has focused on nutritional therapy since his days in medical school in the late 1960s, when he embarked on a personal exploration of the effect of diet on health.

Over the past thirty years, through a combination of nutritional medical therapies, environmental medicine, and traditional acupuncture, he has successfully treated thousands of patients with the illnesses of maladaptation that include obesity, fatigue, chronic pain, headaches, allergies, digestive disorders, asthma, arthritis, anxiety, and depression.

Dr. Moss attended the State University of New York at Buffalo School of Medicine and completed a residency in preventive medicine and family practice at the University of Arizona School of Medicine in 1978. While in Tucson he developed the first holistic health course in the United States for medical students and residents.

In 1978 he established one of the first holistic health medical clinics in the United States. The La Jolla Clinic of Integrative Medicine is the oldest practice of its kind in San Diego. His unique approach to stress induced and chronic medical problems has attracted patients from all over the United States, Mexico, and Europe. The clinic was the subject of the book *Caring and Responsibility* by June Lowenberg, PhD, published in 1989. She researched the groundbreaking methods that he employed as a model for holistic health practice. This book is used as a text in several universities in departments of health policy studies.

Dr. Moss utilizes traditional Five Element acupuncture in his practice. He studied with J. R. Worsley in England in the 1970s and was the first American physician to combine the Five Element system with other areas of holistic health practices. He was an instructor at the UCLA School of Medicine Medical Acupuncture for Physicians postgraduate program, and in 1988 founded the Five Element Acupuncture Physician Training Program, which has trained physicians from throughout the United States and several foreign countries.

Dr. Moss is board certified in medical acupuncture, environmental medicine, and family practice, and is a fellow of both the American Academy of Environmental Medicine and the American Academy of Medical Acupuncture. He has served on the board of directors of the American Academy of Medical Acupuncture, the American Academy of Environmental Medicine, and the American Board of Medical Acupuncture. He is a member of the American Academy of Anti-Aging Medicine, the American Medical Association, and the American College for Advancement in Medicine.

In addition to *The Adaptation Diet*, Dr. Moss is the author of *Power of the Five Elements; The Chinese Medicine Path to Healthy Aging and Stress Resistance*, which details how to improve adaptation and maintain health through knowledge of a person's unique Five Element adaptation type and mind body medicine.

Dr. Moss resides in San Diego County with his wife. His two sons live in Southern California. He continues to practice in La Jolla and teach physicians at medical conferences throughout the United States and abroad.

Contents

Acknowledgments

Over the course of my practice experience, I have learned more about stress and diet from my patients than from any book or medical conference. I am indebted to their commitment to improve their lives through the ideas presented in this book.

I have had many colleagues over the past thirty years who have shared their own clinical experiences and helped me to refine my approach with patients. A partial list includes Jonathan Wright, MD, Jeffrey Bland, PhD, Theron Randolph, MD, Doris Rapp, MD, David Buscher, MD, as well as other members of my professional organizations: the American Academy of Environmental Medicine, the American College for Advancement in Medicine, the Institute for Functional Medicine, and the American Academy of Medical Acupuncture.

I want to thank Kate Jordan and Kathy Sartain for their professional help in organizing this information and making this book possible.

Preface

When I started my practice in integrative medicine in 1978, there was no organized teaching about the impact that nutrition had on well-being and very little understanding of the connection between diet and disease. There were no roadmaps on how to practice nutritional medicine—the field was wide open for physicians like myself to find a way to use diet to make a difference in people's lives. Over the years, practicing this new type of medicine has brought its share of challenges but also incredible satisfaction and excitement.

One of the keys to practicing nutritional medicine was the physician's willingness to suggest to people that they make significant dietary changes and utilize non-pharmaceutical approaches including herbs, antioxidants, vitamins, and minerals to help them recover from illness. Most importantly, the careful observation of the effect of these therapies and the feedback from my patients taught me what was useful and effective. Whenever I found significant improvement in symptoms like fatigue, joint and muscle pain, digestion, allergies, arthritis, headaches, or other conditions either diagnosed or mysterious, I took notice. I wanted to understand why people got better, even if medical research could not explain these beneficial effects and traditional medical therapies were of little use.

In the 1980s, the field of psychoneuroimmunolgy revolutionized the understanding of the mind body connection. Studies showed that beliefs and attitudes are directly linked to chronic medical conditions like heart disease and cancer. This new information made me more aware of the impact that stress can have on health. I began to research how diet and nutrients can impact the function of the brain and the hormonal system, which control the production of stress hormones.

Recent breakthroughs further clarified the changes that can occur in the midbrain, the area of the brain that directly controls stress-hormone secretions. Concepts such as allostasis and allostatic load helped to explain why so many people have trouble recovering their health after stressful experiences and prolonged poor dietary habits. These ideas helped me to appreciate the widespread effect of stress on my patients' symptoms and led me to focus on methods to improve adaptation. I realized that adaptation and reduction of the damage from stress were not just about triggers such as emotional and social situations, but the subtle biochemical stress of poor diets and unhealthy lifestyles. This new information further refined my approach with patients and led to the information in this book.

The Adaptation Diet is the result of working with thousands of patients over the past thirty years, a culmination of what I have learned about regaining adaptation and preventing disease. Especially in today's stressful climate, everyone needs to reduce stress in the areas that they can control. The place to start is at the dinner table.

July 10, 2009
La Jolla, CA

Chapter One
Adaptation and Health

The ability to adapt to changing circumstances is critical to maintaining health and aging well, and this defines the healthy person. Adaptation requires the right set of physical, emotional, and spiritual tools to manage stress and the challenges that life has in store for everyone. My patients that adapt well stay healthy; those that don't are at greater risk for major disease. Often overlooked is the critical effect diet has on the biochemistry of adaptation. In my practice over the past thirty years, I have found that eating habits and nutritional therapies play an enormous role in a patient's capacity for adaptation by keeping his or her body's chemistry better balanced and preventing excessive production of stress hormones from inappropriate dietary practices.

The biochemistry of adaptation starts in the brain and especially the midbrain, the center of control over production of stress hormones: cortisol from the adrenal glands and epinephrine from the adrenals and autonomic nervous system. Hans Selye, the father of modern stress research, identified the three stages of the stress response: alarm, adaptation, and exhaustion or maladaptation. (Selye originally described this third stage as exhaustion because of his initial findings that the adrenal gland no longer produces adequate amounts of cortisol after chronic stress. Later research found that this is often not the case, so a more accurate term for the third stage is maladaptation.) In acute stress, such as a car accident or other threat to survival, the body immediately responds with the alarm reaction, secreting epinephrine (adrenalin) from the adrenal gland and norepinephrine (noradrenalin) from the brain and adrenals. Sweaty palms, increased heart rate, hypervigelence, and rapid breathing prepare the fight-or-flight response to ensure survival reflecting the activity of the sympathetic nervous system. Though often described as short lived and occurring only in the context of immediate life-or-death situations, I have observed many of my patients remaining in this stage chronically, leading to enormous discomfort and anxiety. Caffeine, excessive intake of processed sugars and grains, as well as other foods that trigger maladaptation contribute to continued and inappropriate production of epinephrine.

1

If stress continues beyond a few minutes, cortisol (from the adrenal glands) is produced to raise blood sugar, move blood to muscles and away from digestion, lower levels of sex hormones, and break down protein stores for energy. If a stressful state continues, it is described as the adaptation stage, since it promotes short-term survival even at the cost of long-term health. The adaptation stage with elevated cortisol levels continues as long as there is the perception of a threat, real of imagined. During this stage, inflammation is suppressed and the immune system is inhibited by increasing cortisol levels. Appetite is often stimulated, and a person is more likely to increase energy consumption in the form of higher caloric intake. Increasing weight and the effect of cortisol on inhibiting insulin's action to bring blood sugar into cells can lead to insulin resistance, a condition that we will see is the starting point for many chronic illnesses. Continued stress eventually leads to the maladaptation stage in which the body starts to break down from the effects of elevated cortisol. The maladaptation stage is marked by immune system suppression, poor wound healing, thinning bones, insulin resistance, loss of muscle mass, weight gain around the midsection, depression and anxiety, poor sleep, and elevated blood pressure—all courtesy of elevated levels of cortisol and epinephrine. Another key negative impact of excess cortisol is the loss of muscle mass from the catabolic effect of this hormone. Research has shown that maintaining a healthy amount of lean muscle mass is the single best prevention against premature aging and diseases such as diabetes and heart disease. This is at the root of premature aging. What I have discovered is that the long-term stress that leads to these dire consequences can arise not only from emotional and situational stress but also from what is eaten on a daily basis.

Cortisol is one of forty stress hormones from the adrenal gland called glucocorticoids. The adrenals sit atop the kidneys and are divided into two areas: the adrenal medulla and adrenal cortex. The medulla produces epinephrine and norepinephrine (noradrenalin) used for immediate fight-or-flight response. The cortex has several zones that produce the glucocorticoids (cortisol) and mineralocorticoids, which regulate electrolytes and fluid balance and impact blood pressure. Along with cortisol, the other key hormones are dehydroepiandrosterone (DHEA) and aldosterone.

Cortisol production is tightly regulated by feedback mechanisms in the midbrain, hypothalamus, and pituitary gland, with rising cortisol shutting down further stimulation of the adrenal glands. This feedback loop is called the hypothalamic-pituitary-adrenal (HPA) axis. However, in a state of continued stress, including the wrong foods or eating habits, the feedback loop between the brain and the adrenal glands' cortisol production breaks down, leading to inappropriate levels of cortisol.

Elevated cortisol, from poor dietary habits or other chronic stress, leads to a change in the brain and endocrine system called allostasis. This revolutionary new concept describes the stress response as not simply a short-term adjustment that eventually returns the body to a preset level of cortisol secretion, but a more permanent change in the control over stress hormone production. Even if the original stressful event has been resolved, a new set point might continue, leading to ongoing excessive cortisol production. The damage that occurs from this new set point of cortisol production is called allostatic load, made even worse by poor dietary habits and nutritional deficiencies. Eventually, the wear and tear of poor adaptation and allostatic load coupled with the brain's fail-safe shut down of chronic cortisol elevation lead to a failure of normal cortisol regulation, inhibiting additional secretion by the adrenal gland. This leads to fatigue, anxiety, depression, poor resistance, and an inability to recover normally from life's challenges.

Table 1: Stages of Stress Response

- The brain experiences or thinks of something stressful.
- An immediate release of norepinephrine and epinephrine from the adrenal medulla and sympathetic nervous system occurs (part of the autonomic nervous system not under voluntary control, originating in the brain and spine and branching out to all organ systems).
- This raises heart rate, blood pressure, and respirations and shunts blood from the digestive tract to the muscles.
- If stress is not resolved immediately, the brain secretes CRH (corticotrophin releasing hormone).
- CRH causes release of ACTH within fifteen seconds and the subsequent release of cortisol from the adrenal glands.
- The pancreas releases glucagon that raises circulating levels of glucose for use by the brain and muscles for energy during the stress.
- Prolactin is released by the pituitary to suppress reproductive activity and reduce testosterone, estrogen, and progesterone.
- Thyroid function and growth hormone production is inhibited.
- Endorphins, enkephalins, and vasopressin are secreted to suppress pain and improve cardiac function.
- If the stress continues, many of these effects become chronic and cause continued alterations in physiology.
- Chronic stress leads to elevated blood glucose, insulin resistance, depressed sexual function, weight gain, suppressed immunity, and elevated blood pressure and heart rate.

Emotional states certainly impact adaptation and cortisol levels as well. The brain, through the limbic lobe (the emotional center), connects emotions and perceptions of the world with the appropriate level of cortisol production and nervous system stimulation. Fear, worry, anxiety, or the anticipation of a stressful experience is enough to trigger the brain to initiate the biochemistry of stress. Poor diet, lack of exercise, and obesity also increase cortisol levels and allostatic load. Many people are more prone to be emotionally stressed because of poor dietary habits, which change the brain's chemistry and reduce their ability to adapt, leading again to more cortisol. Even more problematic is the fact that elevated cortisol itself alters the emotional stress response, increasing allostatic load, obesity, and disease.

One of the consequences of chronic cortisol elevation is the impact on how stressful events are perceived. The emotional memory of any significant trauma or stress, whether from a car accident, abuse in a relationship, or any other chronically stressful situation, is stored in two parts of the midbrain (as well as the cerebral cortex): the amygdala and the hippocampus. The memory in the amygdala is implicit and nonspecific, a remembrance that stress occurred, but not of the details of the specific event. When stress continues over time, the amygdala literally grows new neuronal connections to ensure the survival of these memories. The identification of new neuronal growth, called long-term potentiation, is a major breakthrough in the understanding of brain function. (Until recently it was believed that no new cell growth could occur in the central nervous system.) The amygdala contributes directly to elevated cortisol levels through secretion of corticotrophin releasing hormone (CRH). Poor diet could also add to the neuropotentiation of the amygdala.

The amygdala has connections to many parts of the brain and is a major source of corticotropin releasing hormone (CRH), which controls secretion of cortisol and epinephrine, impacting both the fight-or-flight response (the initial reaction to danger and stress) and later allostasis. In addition, the amygdala sends neurons to the sympathetic nervous system to further activate the fight-or-flight response (rapid heart rate, shallow breathing, hypervigilance). Most importantly, it sends "emotional" information to the frontal cortex, which colors perceptions of events and memories, allowing past trauma to influence the present.

Repeated stressful events lead to long-term neuropotentiation in the amygdala, creating increased levels of neurotransmitter chemicals and new growth of neurons that reinforce the stressful memories. However, the implicit memories associated with the amygdala are not necessarily associated with specific events or people, but contain a nonspecific and preconscious response, which often involves fear or other stressful emotions. It is because of the generality and vagueness of this type of memory that the amygdala is so often involved in maladapted chronic stress response. This is part of why people have trouble disengaging themselves from their illness and their stress; the memories and connections from the amygdala keep the stress going, though the details might be lost and perceptions altered. This is at the root of poor adaptation.

The other part of the midbrain that is involved with memories of stressful events is the hippocampus, also a major player in controlling cortisol and epinephrine output. The hippocampus is the seat of declarative memory, a detailed and specific recollection of actual stressful events. The hippocampus is also the site of the regulatory mechanism that measures cortisol levels and influences adrenal secretion of this hormone. Unfortunately, elevated levels of cortisol actually damage the hippocampal neurons, impair long-term potentiation in this part of the midbrain, and degrade the declarative memory.

We are left with an enhanced preconscious and implicit, nonspecific stress memory and response from the amygdala, while lacking the accurate conscious and declarative memory of the hippocampus to modify the stress response. Over time, with ongoing stress, the nonspecific memory of the amygdala gets more entrenched while the details of what the stress actually was, stored in the hippocampus, are lost. This keeps one from being in the present. Although specific memories may not be accessible, perceptions continue to be colored by past events, continuing the stress response.

Long-term stress, whether from situational issues, emotional challenges, or poor dietary habits, can lead to maladaptation and damage from allostatic load through these changes in the brain. Cortisol and CRH from the amygdala are the chemicals that produce these changes. In studies of depressed patients, the hippocampus is 10 to 20 percent smaller, the result of elevated cortisol production. Stress inhibits new neuron formation in the hippocampus that impacts the cortisol control mechanism and declarative memory.

Another outcome of long-term dysregulation of cortisol is the depletion of norepinephrine levels in the brain (especially in an area called the locus coeruleus, which is involved with attentiveness and activity). This is another aspect of the connection between stress and depression (along with the depletion of serotonin and dopamine from the frontal cortex of the brain, which is also caused by elevated cortisol levels). In fact, in animal studies, stress-induced elevated cortisol during pregnancy has been shown to affect the fetus by reducing the size and structure of the hippocampus as the offspring become adults. This could begin to explain why family traits of depression are frequently found. So many of my patients with stress-related medical problems come from dysfunctional families, often with depressed or anxious mothers who did not create a safe and nourishing environment for their children. It's possible that these early experiences affected the midbrain, increasing the vulnerability for stress-induced illness.

These changes in the midbrain explain why some people develop chronic anxiety, depression, or post-traumatic stress disorder. It is now recognized that with treatment—psychotherapy, acupuncture, and possibly medication— the amygdala can remodel and reduce the chronic stimulation of CRH and cortisol. What has been overlooked is the effect of diet and food choices on the biochemistry of stress.

Poor dietary choices—whether they are excessive processed sugars and carbohydrates, inflammation-causing fats, or chemicals in the food chain in nonorganic vegetables, fruits, and proteins—impact cell signaling and increase biochemical stress. This then leads to a greater cortisol response and all its negative consequences. Like emotional traumas or physical illness, daily choices about what is on the dinner plate are a major trigger for increased allostatic load, enhanced amygdala neuropotentiation, and the slippery slope of stress-induced chronic disease.

Cortisol and other stress hormones, which are essential for survival and adaptation to stress, become just as dangerous as the external threats themselves when they are chronically elevated and maladapted. Cortisol levels also increase with age, unlike all other hormones, leading some to call it the 'death hormone' because of its connection to so many degenerative diseases. Cortisol imbalance can lead to fatigue, weight gain, immune suppression, and susceptibility to colds and flu, joint pains, mood swings, anxiety, depression, insomnia, and digestive symptoms such as reflux and heartburn. These symptoms are a message of poor adaptation, not necessarily a message to take antidepressants, stomach acid blockers or pain medication! (See table 2.) Because people often ignore the real meaning of these common complaints, we are in an epidemic of diseases of maladaptation, such as cancer, heart disease, hypertension, stroke, diabetes, Alzheimer's disease, depression, anxiety, and premature aging.

Table 2: Markers of Allostatic Load

- Abdominal obesity, increased waist/hip ratio
- Fatigue
- Elevated blood pressure or pulse
- Poor concentration and memory
- Poor resistance to infections
- Elevated blood sugar, cholesterol, LDL
- Inflammation including headaches, muscle pain, joint pain
- Digestive symptoms, reflux

Increased levels of cortisol have many physiologic costs. Energy is required to deal with a stressor whether it's running from a tiger, dealing with your obnoxious neighbor, or eating a hot dog and chips. Energy is mobilized from storage sites in the body resulting in an increase of glucose, proteins, and fats in the blood to fuel the muscles. The increase in glucose and free fat production can lead to insulin resistance, a state in which insulin (which is needed to bring blood sugar into cells) is not effective because of changes in the cell membrane receptors triggered by elevated cortisol. Cortisol directly contributes to increased glucose levels, leading to more insulin resistance. This leads to a greater risk of heart disease, cancer, and diabetes.

Cortisol is a major trigger for obesity. Increased cortisol levels promote appetite and food-seeking behavior. Cortisol elevation is strongly linked to abdominal fat accumulation, reduced muscle mass, and increased weight. In addition, fat cells in the abdomen have an enzyme that converts inactive to active cortisol to begin a vicious cycle of stress and poor diet causing elevated cortisol, which leads to more fat deposition, which leads to higher cortisol and even more abdominal obesity. For many people, insomnia, depression, anxiety, and fatigue—all symptoms made worse or initiated by cortisol dysregulation—are linked to excessive caloric intake and obesity.

Elevated cortisol also inhibits thyroid function further adding to weight gain and fatigue. The immune system is suppressed in a variety of ways by excess cortisol, leading to a greater chance for serious infections, causing more maladaptation. It has also been linked to bone loss, lowered sex hormones, and greater inflammation.

Elevated stress hormones inhibit digestion and have been associated with ulcers, intestinal disorders, and irritable bowel syndrome (a condition of abdominal pain, bloating, and alternating diarrhea and constipation). With these and other stress-induced digestive problems, poor functioning of the small intestine and colon can lead to malabsorption of nutrients and nutritional deficiencies. The resulting nutritional deficiencies open the door to many other medical problems, worsening maladaptation and allostatic load.

Table 3: Early Signs of Maladaptation

Emotional and behavioral signs	Physical signs and symptoms
• Fatigue	• Weight gain esp. in abdomen
• Nervousness	• Hypoglycemia, low blood sugar
• Anxiety, agitation	• Headaches
• Little resilience, stress intolerance	• Frequent colds and flu
• Noise sensitivity	• Muscular pain and tenderness

- Worries and fears
- Inability to concentrate
- Alcohol craving or intolerance
- Crave sweets and fats
- Lower sex drive

- Joint pain and tenderness
- Heart palpitations, elevated heart rate
- Menstrual irregularity
- Back or neck pain
- Abdominal discomfort

Table 4: Later Signs and Symptoms of Maladaptation

- Poor wound healing
- Increased blood pressure
- Apathy
- Feel life is difficult, unfair
- Salt craving
- Worsening premenstrual tension
- Generalized weakness
- Poor memory
- Loss of bone density (osteoporosis)

- Allergies
- Sexual dysfunction, impotency
- Loss of muscle mass
- Depression
- Facial swelling, fluid retention
- Glucose (sugar) intolerance, insulin resistance
- Moon (swollen) face

The key to adaptation and control over cortisol through diet is threefold: 1) reducing inflammation through healthy food choices, including the use of good fats, 2) preventing insulin resistance and metabolic syndrome through the use of low-glycemic-index carbohydrates and organically grown whole food, and 3) identifying and avoiding food allergies to reduce many nagging symptoms and decrease cortisol production. This book describes in detail the dietary changes needed to achieve normal cortisol levels and improve the biochemistry of adaptation, reduce allostatic load, and reduce the likelihood of premature aging. Following these guidelines has helped many of my patients achieve adaptation, lose weight, and improve well-being.

Chapter Two
Food and Adaptation

During my thirty years of practice, I have seen the remarkable effects diet can have on stress and regulating cortisol levels. I first became aware of the impact of diet on health when I was in medical school in the late 1960s. What I learned came not from my professors (in 1969 there was no instruction on nutrition; even today there still is little taught) but from personal research my classmates and I performed. I had been eating a standard American diet (SAD) heavy on meat, cheese, bread, and sweets. It left me a bit overweight and very sluggish. When my roommates and I decided to adopt a macrobiotic diet (a Westernized application of a traditional Oriental diet popularized by Michio Kushi), my life changed.

Our version of the macrobiotic diet included brown rice, cooked vegetables, tofu, fish, and chicken. There was no red meat, sweets, fruits or sweeteners, dairy, corn, or wheat. The results were remarkable—I lost weight effortlessly, my energy improved, I was more relaxed, and I felt mentally sharper. Aches and pains disappeared, and my digestion improved as well. It was then that my orientation toward what I was being taught in medical school changed. I realized, as Hippocrates had said, that food is your best medicine, and I would have to teach myself how best to help my patients. My practice today is consistent with that personal epiphany in 1969.

Current research demonstrates convincingly that diet contributes to 35 percent of all cancers and the majority of heart disease. The standard American diet not only is implicated in these chronic diseases, it is the biggest factor in premature aging. Not appreciated, however, is the mechanism by which diet directly causes maladaptation and cortisol dysregulation. To counteract the maladaptive effects of eating habits, I developed the Adaptation Diet, a template to regain adaptation and robust health. Every aspect of the Adaptation Diet is aimed at cortisol regulation and reduction of allostatic load, leading to weight loss, enhanced well-being, and disease prevention.

Food and Adaptation

Shane looked at me in disbelief. He was a strapping man in his midforties with wide-open eyes that made him appear as if he had just been startled. His main complaints were insomnia, anxiety, and a mind that raced like a NASCAR driver. Luckily, he had not yet developed any heart disease or diabetes. I had measured his salivary cortisol levels, and they were off the chart. He was expecting me to reach for my prescription pad; instead I told him that if he wanted to eliminate his problems, he needed to normalize his cortisol and the place to begin was in changing what he ate.

I recommended that Shane stop eating all processed foods: white flour products, and most importantly, all sugar, desserts, candy, and other sweets. He was put on a program to keep his blood sugar stable throughout the day by having a protein-rich breakfast and snacks of nuts, seeds, nut butter, or protein powder. In six weeks, he repeated his cortisol test. He came in to my office soon thereafter, his demeanor drastically changed. He sat calmly in his chair, not fidgeting and able to focus on what I was saying.

Within a week of changing his diet, Shane was sleeping better, he was calmer, and most surprising to him, he felt more positive about life in general. Over the next six weeks, he started to feel like his old self, was more pleasant to be around (according to his wife), and was more productive at work. His salivary cortisol levels had come down to normal.

Another patient, Beth, had just completed her food allergy skin testing when she saw me for a consultation. She was distinctly overweight, fatigued, irritable (especially the week prior to her menstrual period), and a poor sleeper. Beth, thirty-two years old, mother of two, felt like she was eighty. Her joints hurt every day, her muscles were weak, and she had no stamina. As a child, Beth had a history of hay fever and a touch of asthma, which she had outgrown. Most of her doctors had assumed she was depressed and treated her with antidepressants, which only made her feel more tired and out of sorts.

Beth looked a bit panicked when we started to talk about her test results. The first words out of her mouth were "What am I going to eat?" Her skin testing revealed significant reactions to wheat, dairy, bakers yeast, corn, and tomatoes. Her cortisol test showed a dramatic deficit in cortisol production, especially in the morning. (She was in the later stages of cortisol dysregulation; after decades of elevated levels, her brain had shut down the cortisol response.). With the help of our nutritionist, we created a well-balanced diet including a small amount of grains other than wheat and corn and the elimination of tomatoes, dairy, and yeast.

It took only a few days for Beth to see the change. The first thing she noticed was that her aches and pains disappeared. Gradually she began to sleep better, was less irritable, and lost some of her extra weight. When I retested her cortisol levels two month later, her morning measurement was in the normal range. She came in after that with a smile as wide as her whole face. She had not felt this good since she was a youngster and thanked me for giving her a chance to be happy again.

What happened for Beth and Shane? They had regained adaptation, reducing their allostatic load, rapidly normalizing their cortisol levels. The foods that Shane ate that caused low blood sugar as well as the unhealthy fats that he was exposed to daily had raised his cortisol into dangerous levels. Yet, within a short period of time, his hypothalamic-pituitary-adrenal (HPA) axis, with help from this change in eating habits, reverted to a normal pattern. In Beth's case, she reduced her inflammatory response by avoiding foods that she was allergic to, allowing her HPA axis to reset normal cortisol levels.

Fortunately, I have been able to help many patients improve their allostatic load simply by making dietary changes. For some, avoiding food allergies is the key. For others, it is maintaining normal blood sugar and avoiding hypoglycemia. For all my patients, a key component is reducing foods that trigger inflammation, such as refined sugar and flour products, fried foods, and animal protein that is not free range or fed organically. (For example, free-range chicken eggs have one tenth of the omega 6 inflammatory fatty acids as industrially produced eggs.)

The common denominator for all these patients is finding a way to regain biochemical adaptation through limiting their body's abnormal cortisol response to the wrong foods. I call this approach the Adaptation Diet because the goal is to control the abnormal production of cortisol and the cascade of hormonal changes that characterize maladaptation.

The components of the Adaptation Diet are:
- Emphasis on anti-inflammatory foods rich in phytonutrients such as flavonoids, carotenoids, and omega 3 fatty acids, and elimination of inflammation-causing foods, especially the pro-inflammatory fats including omega 6 fatty acids and trans fats
- Identifying food allergies and avoiding allergy-causing foods
- Avoidance of gluten-containing grains if gluten sensitive
- Use of low-glycemic-index carbohydrates, maintenance of normal blood sugar and insulin levels, and avoidance of hypoglycemia and insulin resistance

- Use of foods, herbs, and supplements that normalize cortisol
- Detoxification to reduce inflammation and cellular damage

There are five aspects of dietary habits that directly link to elevated cortisol levels. The first is food composition. Studies have shown that high intake of protein and fat (especially the "wrong" fats) and simple carbohydrates increases cortisol production significantly in stressful situations. On the other hand, consumption of whole grains and omega 3 fatty acids can lower the cortisol response. In a study performed by Markus (published in *Physiology Behavior,* 2000), people identified as high stress responders (you probably know if you are in that category) showed lower cortisol responses and less depression when fed a complex-carbohydrate-rich and protein-poor diet as compared to a typical high-protein diet. (The protein in this study was not defined and probably contained excessive amounts of red meat, dairy, and eggs. If the protein was mainly fish and vegetable based, cortisol levels would not have been adversely affected.)

The second key to lower cortisol is maintaining normal blood sugar and avoiding spikes in insulin production that can lead to insulin resistance. Insulin resistance is an increasingly common finding in overweight individuals. In insulin resistance, the receptors on the cell surface become dysfunctional, leading to the production of more and more insulin. Inflammation is thought to be one cause of this cell membrane dysfunction. Repeated use of refined sugars and simple carbohydrates can lead to metabolic syndrome (high blood pressure, elevated blood fats and increased risk for heart disease), obesity, and diabetes.

High-glycemic index (a measure of how rapidly a food causes a spike in blood sugar) and   refined and processed foods such as white flour products, (white bread, cookies, pastas, candy, muffins), refined sugar, juices with added sugar, soft drinks, most breakfast cereals, and chips are the main culprits in poor control of blood sugar. Using foods that are high in fiber slows digestion of carbohydrates and improves blood sugar maintenance, preventing blood sugar spikes, increased insulin production leading to obesity, and hypoglycemia. Beans, brown rice, steel-cut oatmeal, buckwheat, and green vegetables like broccoli and spinach are some of the good sources of fiber.

Another concern regarding high-glycemic-index meals is the impact they have on appetite and eating behavior. Since low blood sugar often follows the spike in glucose from high-glycemic foods, eating behavior is enhanced and people will consume more calories throughout the day after a high-glycemic meal. This is a setup for weight gain, abdominal obesity, and eventually insulin resistance and all its subsequent heath risks.

On a flight recently, I listened carefully to the list of drinks and snacks that were offered to the passengers. As I watched the majority of my seatmates consume sodas, juice, crackers, and other high-glycemic-index foods, it wasn't hard to imagine what was happening to their physiology and allostatic load while they silently flew toward their destination. The blast of sugar triggered a spike in blood glucose, triggering a potent release of insulin to drive the glucose into the cells, which then led to hypoglycemia and a release of the counter-regulatory hormones, including cortisol. This soft-drink-induced event ended with release of free fatty acids in the form of triglycerides and other fats and increased adiposity in the abdominal cavity.

Repeated sodas later, the sequence changes. No longer does the insulin effectively bring down the glucose from the sudden burst of sugar, because insulin resistance has occurred. The adipocytes (fat cells) inflammatory hormones including resisten that interfere with the cell membrane signaling from the insulin, preventing the cell from mobilizing the mechanism that takes in glucose from the bloodstream for energy. The result is more allostatic load, cortisol, free fats, obesity, and inflammation. The cycle repeats with every high-glycemic meal leading to first being overweight with a body mass index (BMI) of 25–30, then obese with a BMI of 30–35, then morbidly obese (over 35 BMI), and finally super morbid obesity with a BMI over 50.

The third key to lower cortisol is choosing the right fats: foods rich in omega 3 and gamma linoleic omega 6 fats. Salmon, walnuts, almonds, halibut, flaxseed, pumpkin seeds, and other sources of these good fats reduce inflammation and prevent excess cortisol production. Avoidance of the omega 6 fats found in vegetable oils, including corn oil, safflower oil, and sunflower oil; the trans fats found in most processed foods; as well as the saturated fats in red meat and whole dairy also lowers inflammation and the demand for cortisol.

The fourth key to lower cortisol is to include foods that are rich in flavonoids, carotenoids, and other phytonutrients that can help to detoxify the body and protect cellular health. Green tea, garlic, onions, red wine, blueberries, broccoli, tomatoes, bell peppers, and kale are just a few of these super foods that reduce the need for cortisol by controlling cellular damage.

The fifth, and most overlooked key in controlling cortisol, is identifying food allergies and intolerance. Reactions from food allergies trigger a dramatic rise in cortisol; in my clinical experience it is one of the most frequent causes of depression, fatigue, anxiety, insomnia, aches and pains, and digestive problems. The most common food triggers are the most commonly overused foods: wheat, beef, yeast, corn, dairy, sugar, and soy.

When I look back at my early experiment with macrobiotics, it amazes me that most of these five keys to lower cortisol were accomplished through that diet. Today I know much more about the mechanisms of food-triggered cortisol response and have helped many of my patients regain adaptation through diet. Let's look at another of my patients with a common story.

Sara was always feeling stressed. She was anxious, light headed, tired, and depressed. No longer able to hold a job, she was in a doctor shopping frenzy. Sara had a history of episodic depression and fatigue as well as hay fever and other allergies. At thirty-six, she felt that life was passing her by, was rarely feeling well, and was always on the verge of overreacting to whatever challenges life presented.

Her complaints made me suspicious of cortisol dysregulation. I ordered a salivary cortisol test that showed highly elevated cortisol levels, typical for someone in a chronically stressed state. Though Sara was well versed in stress-management techniques, including meditation and exercise, it did her little good. What did matter was her diet.

Every day when waking, her level of dread and anxiety was at its highest, calming down after breakfast. Sara had always had an enormous sweet tooth; her breakfast was usually a sweet roll, juice, and coffee. She snacked on chips and pretzels throughout the day. She also liked red meat; one of her favorites was a carne asada burrito at a local Mexican fast-food restaurant. Without knowing it, Sara had multiple food allergies that we later identified though intradermal skin testing. This technique involves placing a small amount of a food antigen under the skin and observing the wheal growth over a period of ten minutes. According to the American Academy of Environmental Medicine, this is the gold standard for food allergy tests.

Sara's diet contributed to elevated cortisol in several different ways. She had reactive hypoglycemia—low blood sugar as a result of eating foods rich in simple sugars and white flour products. Sara felt so dreadful in the morning because her late-night desserts first caused a spike in her blood sugar and insulin, then a dip, triggering a compensatory response to raise her blood sugar levels back up. The hormones that accomplish this include cortisol and norepinephrine. As a result of this all-night hormonal chaos, she awoke with anxiety. (One of cortisol's roles is to elevate blood sugar if it drops too low from excess insulin production, often the result of eating processed foods.)

Throughout the day, Sara's blood sugar would bounce up and down—her simple-carbohydrate-rich breakfast and lunch (a sandwich and some chips) led to low blood sugar in the midafternoon and additional increases in cortisol and norepinephrine. She would feel tired, out of sorts, thick headed with poor concentration, anxious, and jittery. (Most people with reactive hypoglycemia have their worst slump after lunch, probably because they eat little at breakfast and lack the right foods at lunch, whereas dinner is typically higher in protein and more substantial.)

Unfortunately, low blood sugar was not the only trigger for Sara's elevated cortisol. Her snacks often included foods with unhealthy omega 6 fats, processed from corn or soy oils, as well as trans fatty acids. These fats trigger cellular inflammation, though there are few signs or warnings that this is occurring. The inflammatory response to these foods is a significant biochemical process affecting the coronary arteries, brain neurons, joints, and the digestive tract. The body's antidote for inflammation is cortisol. The chips, pretzels, cookies, and fast foods create a clarion call to the adrenal glands to help rescue the body from the onslaughts of the modern food industry.

One more factor contributing to Sara's medley of cortisol triggers was food allergy. Sara had a history of respiratory allergies from her teenage years, a hint that food allergies were playing a role. She had other signs including digestive complaints, fatigue, headaches, and dizziness, all occurring after meals. When she avoided the foods we eventually identified as her triggers—corn, soy, wheat, and dairy—she improved quickly.

Here's what Sara needed to do to resolve the cortisol overload from her diet:
1) To improve her hypoglycemia:
   • Eat a protein-rich breakfast (choose from eggs, low-fat unsweetened yogurt, oatmeal, nut butter, nuts, seeds, fish); use only complex carbohydrates (whole grains, especially steel-cut oatmeal); avoid all high-glycemic index foods (see appendix section 1)
   • Have protein snacks between breakfast and lunch, and lunch and dinner (nuts, seeds, nut butter, beans, unsweetened yogurt, turkey, chicken, fish)
   • Avoid all processed sweets, white sugar, white flour, processed grains, and fruit-sweetened food and drinks—use whole fruit as dessert
   • Supplement with protein powder as needed between meals or as a meal replacement (when in a rush)
   • Avoid sweets late at night—use complex carbohydrates and protein instead

2) To improve the types of fatty acids in her diet:
   - Avoid snack foods such as pretzels, chips, cookies
   - Never use margarine, corn oil, or polyunsaturated oils
   - Use olive, grape seed, or canola oil for cooking or salad dressing
   - Avoid fried foods, especially deep-fried fast foods
   - Increase intake of wild salmon, avocadoes, walnuts, almonds, flaxseed (powder and oil), halibut
   - Decrease red meat intake; use only low-fat dairy
   - Never use trans fats
3) To improve the food allergies:
   - Follow the avoidance and challenge program of the Adaptation Diet to identify the main food triggers
   - If she has access to a physician experienced in food allergy management, get skin tested or blood tests that are approved by the American Academy of Environmental Medicine
   - If not sure about which foods are triggers, avoid the big seven of delayed food allergy: wheat, corn, soy, dairy, yeast, beef, and sugar.
   - Adopt a rotation diet, eating foods no more often than twice a week that are causing symptoms

Once these suggestions were adopted, Sara improved quickly. Her cortisol levels returned to normal. She slept more deeply and awoke refreshed. Her anxiety and fatigue during the day were much reduced. She was thrilled by a weight loss of twelve pounds over six weeks.

As many of my patients have proven, what is on the dinner plate has as much an influence on adaptation and aging well as anything else that a person can control. Cortisol production increases when there is inflammation from the wrong fats in the diet, hypoglycemia in response to eating high-glycemic foods, food allergy reactions, increased abdominal girth and insulin resistance, and exposure to toxins. If you think these triggers are not common in the American diet, you are wrong. Obesity rates are now nearing 50 percent of all Americans, including children. Food allergies and intolerance affect nearly that many. Inflammation is the result of eating the wrong fats—omega 6 instead of omega 3 (packaged and processed foods, meat, eggs, and whole-fat dairy instead of cold-water fish, walnuts, almonds) as well as the result of exposure to pollutants in the food chain.

The Adaptation Diet is the answer to adaptation and aging well. Most Americans' eating habits contribute to premature aging through triggers that raise cortisol levels. Perhaps we should rename the standard American diet the Maladaptation diet, because most people are doing themselves harm by increasing their stress hormones through their dietary habits.

Chapter Three
Detoxification and Adaptation

The first step of the Adaptation Diet program in reclaiming adaptation is a three-week detoxification program to assist the body's ability to remove toxins and pollutants and reduce allostatic load. The concept of detoxification goes back to Hippocrates, considered the founder of Western medicine, who believed that cleanliness was key to health and advocated fasting, steam baths, bathing in springs, and gymnastics. The Chinese Taoist physicians also were aware of the need to detoxify, employing herbal remedies to clear poisons from the system. Detoxification primarily occurs through the liver, kidney, and digestive tract. The liver, the principal organ of detoxification, converts toxic chemicals, drugs, hormones, and products of metabolism such as free radicals, to inert substances that can be eliminated through the gut or the kidneys.

Repeatedly, my patients have dramatic improvements in a host of symptoms by simply "cleaning up" their diets during the detox phase. Headaches, joint pains, constipation, or abdominal discomfort and fatigue are just a few of the problems that consistently begin to resolve, often within the first ten days of the program. Symptoms improve because of the use of more nutritious foods, the avoidance of simple sugars and starches and other toxic foods, the elimination of the foods that are most likely to trigger an allergic response, and the improvement in the detoxification pathways to clear chemicals and other toxins from the body. All of these aspects have one thing in common: the normalization of the cortisol response.

Modern life presents an enormous challenge to the detoxification system. For example, to make shelf life longer, a Twinkies cake has thirty-nine ingredients including polysorbate 60 replacing real cream, artificial vanillin instead of the real thing, diacetyl instead of butter, and yellow no. 5 and red no. 40 for coloring. In addition are industrial chemicals such as corn dextrin used as a thickener (and also used in glues) and calcium sulfate or food-grade plaster of Paris. The shelf life of a cake made with only natural ingredients would be a few days; the shelf life of a Twinkie is many months if not years.

The food industry, to meet the demands of the American diet, has loaded the average American with thousands of chemicals, every one of which needs to be detoxified. Though alone each of these chemicals are not necessarily toxic, when combined with unintentional additives to the food chain such as pesticide residues, and industrial chemicals found in air and water pollution, any breakdown in the detoxification system, from stress or poor nutritional status, can lead to disastrous results and biochemical maladaptation.

Annually, almost one billion pounds of pesticides are sprayed on food crops in the United States. The average American consumes one gallon of food additives a year. There are also over 10,000 incidental additives found in the food chain including pesticides, fumigants, solvents, colorings, stimulants, chlorine bleach, and plastic polymers. In 1970, the FDA began assessing the problem of chemicals in the food chain. Through a combination of lack of funding and a lack of political will because of industry economic influences, the FDA created the Generally Regarded as Safe list, consisting of chemicals that were never studied but were assumed to be safe. Twenty-seven hundred chemicals were placed on this list in 1970, and the number of untested chemicals has continued to grow since.

Similar to assumptions made about environmental chemicals, chemicals in the food chain were allowed if they did not prove to be carcinogenic, even if there were other effects on the immune system. In the few chemicals that were studied, no additive effects of the chemicals were looked for. For example, when a study showed a minority of animals became ill, but most were not affected, the chemical was deemed safe. This translates into millions of people being at risk from the additive effects of the thousands of chemicals in the food chain. To survive this onslaught of man-made chemicals, the detoxification system must be operating efficiently. Unfortunately, the detoxification process requires adequate intake of phytonutrients, sorely lacking in the typical American diet.

It is not just the food chain that provides challenges to the detoxification system. The Environmental Protection Agency estimated that over 2 billion pounds of toxic chemicals are released annually into the environment in the United States. Six hundred pounds of air pollution was released for every person in America per year. There are over 65,000 chemical compounds in use in the United States, and only 1,200, or less than 2 percent, have been adequately studied. Of those that were studied, the only tests done looked for carcinogenicity and not other subtle effects on the immune system and allostatic load.

Table 1: Classes of Toxins

- Airborne industrial chemicals and combustion pollutants (includes PCBs, halogenated hydrocarbons that are airborne)
- Pesticides—over 800 different chemicals including herbicides, fungicides, insecticides
- Endocrine disruptors such as DDT and PCB; phthallates in plastic; synthetic steroids in meats and poultry
- Toxic metals including lead, mercury, cadmium, and arsenic, which accumulate in the body and are difficult to remove
- Food additives, preservatives, and drugs found intentionally and inadvertently in food and water

The Detoxification System

Diets rich in phytonutrients support detoxification by providing cofactors for the liver to convert toxins to inert materials. The liver does this through two steps: Phase One deactivates the toxic substance through the cytochrome P450 pathway, and Phase Two clears the toxin by linking with another compound through either conjugation, sulfation, methylation, or acetylation. Once this occurs, the chemical is removed through the kidney or colon.

These reactions are dependent on adequate supplies of nutrients such as B vitamins, glutathione, amino acids, flavonoids and phospholipids, essential amino acids, zinc, copper, selenium, Coenzyme Q10, vitamins A, C, E, and other plant-derived nutrients. Proper functioning of both phases of detoxification is needed to avoid the buildup of intermediate metabolites that can cause free radical damage to cell membranes. The activities of the Phase One and Phase Two systems have to be coordinated, otherwise an excess or deficiency of one versus the other can lead to significant medical problems.

The body protects against free radicals and oxidant damage through the action of antioxidants. Some of the key antioxidants are made by the body and include uric acid, albumin, and bilirubin. The body, however, can only produce a small portion of the required antioxidants, which otherwise must come from the diet. The key food-based antioxidants are vitamin C, vitamin E, carotenoids (vitamin A, beta carotene, lycopene, lutein), selenium, zinc, coenzyme Q10, bioflavonoids, manganese, molybdenum, copper, and sulfur. These antioxidants work in concert with each other, and high doses of one without the others can be counterproductive.

The intestine is also an organ of detoxification. It is estimated that over twenty-five tons of food are processed over a lifetime with exposure to a large number of xenobiotics (chemicals that destroy good bacteria) and antigens in the digestive tract. Detoxification enzymes are found in the wall of the intestine to reduce the toxic load of the body. Beneficial bacteria in the gut such as acidophilus and bifidus also are protective. Reducing the good bacteria levels in the intestines from antibiotics or other medications allows overgrowth of unhealthful bacteria that undo the Phase Two reactions and allow reabsorption of toxic substances into the body, furthering the toxic load, creating inflammation, and elevating cortisol production.

Problems with the barrier function of the intestines will also lead to increased toxin load. The so-called leaky gut, or increased intestinal permeability, is the result of poor nutrition, stress, poor oxygenation, and medications such as antibiotics which can lead to overgrowth of *Candida albicans,* a yeast organism responsible for vaginitis in women and digestive symptoms such as bloating and generalized fatigue. A "leaky gut" increases absorption of toxins and food allergens leading to a host of inflammatory states and higher cortisol levels.

Nutritional support of the detoxification process involves specific foods and nutrients that are required for Phase One and Phase Two of the process. Phase One detoxification involves the cytochrome P450 enzyme system found in the mitochondria (a small organelle inside the cell that is involved in energy production). The end product of Phase One detoxification is often free radicals, which are products of oxidation (combustion) of the toxic substances and are themselves injurious to the cell. They include singlet oxygen, peroxides, and other charged molecules. When free radicals come in contact with cells, they can damage the mitochondria and cause deficiency in the energy production of the cells as well as neuromuscular problems.

Free radicals can injure any organ in the body, especially the liver. The exposure of the cell nucleus to free radicals can alter the genetic code of the cell and be a precursor to cancer. The creation of these toxic intermediates in the detoxification process is influenced by a number of factors including the use of medications. Certain drugs such as the acid blockers Zantac, Pepcid, Tagamet; antidepressants including fluoxetine, paroxetene, norfluoxetene, sertraline; antibiotics such as erythromycin, Biaxin, and fluoroquinilones; and antifungals including Nizoral, Diflucan, and Sporonox inhibit the cytochrome system from detoxifying other medications. Another over-the-counter medication that depletes the sulfur compounds needed for detoxification is acetaminophen, found in Tylenol and other medications. The Phase One process can be dangerous if inhibited by drugs or by creating excessive amounts of free radicals, which cannot be converted to nontoxic substances.

Toxins (urea, lactic acid, and others) are also produced from normal metabolism and require detoxification by the liver. Hormones including estrogen, testosterone, thyroid, and especially cortisol require detoxification by the liver, a process that can be compromised by chemical toxins called xenohormones, which mimic the body's own hormones. With excess accumulation of inorganic chemicals, it is possible that hormones themselves become a source of toxicity. Poor dietary habits, nutritional deficiencies, and inadequate intake of protein and carbohydrates can compromise the detoxification pathways, leading to a progressive buildup of toxins and the consequence of greater biochemical stress.

Table 2: Symptoms of Inadequate Detoxification

- Fatigue and malaise
- Cognitive problems such as poor concentration, memory loss
- Depression and anxiety
- Musculoskeletal symptoms such as fibromyalgia, muscle aches, arthritis
- Sensitivity to odors and medications
- Parasthesias or tingling and nerve problems in the extremities
- Edema and fluid retention
- Worsening symptoms after anesthesia or pregnancy
- Multiple allergies to foods, molds, pollens

Food choices also make a difference in the detoxification of toxins. A diet rich in vegetables, fruits, nuts, seeds, legumes, whole grains, and seafood reduces the toxic effect of pesticides and carcinogens and over-the-counter drugs. However, proteins that are pro-inflammatory with high levels of arachidonic acid (red meat, pork, dairy, eggs), or other unhealthy fats (fried foods, trans fats in baked goods) generate greater toxic loads on the liver. High-glycemic foods including white flour and processed sugars can depress the P450 system, as well as increase the prostaglandins and leukotrienes that generate more free radical stress. Good fats such as omega 3 fatty acids from fish and walnuts, and monounsaturated from olive oil, grapeseed oil, almonds, and avocadoes are helpful in the detoxification process.

Increased fiber intake benefits detoxification in many ways. Fiber promotes the removal of conjugated toxins (from Phase Two) that are excreted in bile into the intestines. Less of these toxins are reabsorbed with adequate dietary fiber. Fiber can directly bind toxins that are mutagens (cause cell mutation and cancer) and remove them from the body. Fiber also supports the growth of beneficial bacteria in the gut that play a significant role in detoxification. These bacteria including lactobacillus and bifidobacter directly detoxify hormones as well as xenobiotics arising from contaminants in the food chain. Improved colon function with adequate fiber goes a long way to detoxifying the whole body.

Table 3: Detoxifying the Diet

- Eat vegetables and fruits grown organically
- Use fiber-rich foods including flaxseed powder, oat and rice bran, and legumes
- Use antibiotic and hormone free meat and chicken and limit red meat to once a week
- Drink only filtered water
- Use only free-range eggs fed on organic feed
- Avoid farm raised fish
- Limit the amount of swordfish, tilefish, tuna, and other fish known to have high mercury levels
- Avoid all foods that are fried or contain trans fatty acids and other unhealthy fats
- Do not use soft drinks or excessive fruit juice
- Restrict caffeine including coffee, black teas
- Eliminate refined sugar including candy, pastries, sweetened canned fruits, ice cream, cookies, cakes
- Use live-culture, unsweetened yogurt or kefir to increase beneficial bacteria

Fasting

Over the centuries therapeutic fasting has been employed as a means to detoxify and purify the body. In my practice, I suggest either a short juice fast, a more extended raw-food diet, or the use of medical foods designed to detoxify while placing less stress on the body. I do not recommend water fasting for my patients because of the severe ketosis (acidosis and protein breakdown) and rapid release of toxins that occur in a starvation mode. Severe caloric restriction also raises cortisol levels in response to stress from inadequate calories. I suggest that any fasting or detoxification be undertaken with medical supervision.

Juice fasting is best if based on organic vegetable juices such as combinations of celery, spinach, carrot, and parsley. Before any fasting or severely restricted diet, it is necessary that you refrain from as many over the counter medications as possible, avoid smoking, and stop all alcohol and caffeine for at least three weeks before undertaking a more restricted program. This avoids a severe detoxification crisis.

It is possible to juice fast one day a week, or possibly three days in a row every four months. I prefer my patients use the medical food approach that is designed to improve the liver's detoxification pathways while restricting the diet and avoiding "offender" foods.

Table 4: The Effect of Food on Adaptation and Longevity: A Short List

- One-quarter cup of nuts eaten five times per week lowers the risk for diabetes 21 percent and reduces LDL cholesterol by one-third
- Five servings of fruits and vegetables per day reduces the incidence of cancer, heart disease, diabetes, hypertension
- Twenty-five grams of fiber per day reduces risk of heart disease (by 30 percent), breast cancer, colon cancer, and stroke
- Intake of omega 3 fatty acids from fish, oleic acid from olive oil, and avoidance of trans fatty acids reduces the risk of heart disease, stroke, and diabetes

All the foods listed in table 4, as well as many others rich in flavonoids, carotenoids, and other phytonutrients, improve detoxification, reduce inflammation, and help maintain healthy levels of cortisol. Despite the enormous number of toxic exposures that are part of modern life, with the right dietary approach, the detoxification system is able to cope. Improved detoxification reduces inflammation, therefore decreasing allostatic load and cortisol production. To begin this journey back to adaptation, a three week detoxification program is helpful to jump-start the process. In my practice, I use a diet that limits the trigger foods that can induce an allergic response and emphasizes foods without additives, chemicals, and toxic fats. In addition, these are foods that are rich in detoxifying and anti-inflammatory phytonutrients. Adding nutritional supplements improves the liver detoxification systems and accelerates the process.

The Adaptation Diet Program is divided into three phases:

<u>Phase One</u>:   Weeks One to Three: Detoxification and elimination of allergens

<u>Phase Two</u>:   Weeks Four and Five: Food allergy challenge

<u>Phase Three</u>:   Week Six On: Maintenance with an anti-inflammatory, low-allergy, phytonutrient-rich, blood-sugar balancing diet.

Most of my patients by week six are feeling better and are on their way to regaining adaptation, losing weight, and reducing cortisol and allostatic load.

Chapter Four

Adaptation Diet Phases One and Two: Detoxification and Identification of Food Allergies

Dietary Detoxification: Weeks One to Three

Surprisingly, the body's ability to detoxify and reduce allostatic load is quickly activated through dietary changes. I have used several diets in my practice to help people detoxify and have found the approach detailed here the easiest to adopt. Success requires a willingness to follow the program precisely. There often is a struggle over giving up desserts, alcohol, coffee, and other comfort foods, however after the first three to four days, most people don't even miss these foods. My patients have shown me that if given a chance, the body will respond and recover from maladaptation.

Any person who has medical issues including diabetes, heart disease, cancer, or any chronic or acute medical condition has to be under the care of a physician before undertaking the detoxification phase of the Adaptation Diet. Withdrawal from alcohol in people who habitually drink can be life threatening and must be closely supervised. Caffeine-withdrawal symptoms are also very common in habitual coffee or tea drinkers. Symptoms often include headaches, fatigue, and irritability. I suggest that caffeine withdrawal be accomplished before starting Phase One of the diet so that no over-the-counter pain medications are required. Some people on an elimination diet for the first time will feel significant symptoms from the detoxification effect and withdrawal from their normal food patterns. Some of my patients feel quite badly during this phase of the program and needed my guidance to adjust how they went through the dietary change. Therefore, any person with health concerns should not attempt this diet unless supervised by their physician.

One of my patients illustrated what can occur with sudden caffeine withdrawal. Benita was a patient with fibromyalgia (severe widespread muscle pain), headaches, and fatigue. Within a week of starting the detoxification diet, she developed major headaches and eye pain. Unfortunately she went to her ophthalmologist without first consulting me. He thought she had developed a problem with her visual system and ordered several tests and treated her with pain medications. Benita, a heavy coffee user, had abruptly stopped her coffee intake resulting in migraine-type headaches from caffeine withdrawal. However, even in the face of the caffeine withdrawal symptoms, her generalized muscle pain and fatigue had greatly improved from removing the toxins in her diet and avoiding her probable food allergy triggers. If Benita had gradually withdrawn from caffeine, her symptoms would have been much less severe and her detoxification would have gone smoothly.

Some people will actually experience withdrawal symptoms from sugars, wheat products, and other food allergens, including headaches, fatigue, and mood changes. These symptoms are typically short lived and generally do not require intervention, though short-term (one or two days) use of acetaminophen or aspirin is allowed if needed. If symptoms of fatigue, severe headaches, or muscle pain continue past the fourth day, the diet should be terminated and a physician consulted.

I suggest starting the detoxification part of the diet over the weekend to prevent symptoms from taking you away from work. Purchase the foods that are included in the diet ahead of time so that you are not tempted to revert to old habits. If you use caffeinated coffee or teas, gradually withdraw from these foods over at least one week before starting the detoxification diet. Make sure to have adequate water intake, at least 64 ounces per day. It is important to use only purified water, either bottled or filtered. Organic foods are best where available. It is especially important that organically raised animal protein is used. Cravings for sweets, starches, and other comfort food will occur for most people, usually resolving within the first four days.

Some people will feel more fatigue during the first week of the diet. It is recommended to cut down on intense exercise and possibly just walk during the first two weeks. If fatigue becomes more intense past the first few days, the diet should be stopped and a health care practitioner consulted.

Table 1 lists the foods to include and those to avoid during the detoxification phase. Introducing foods that are not on the allowed list will slow down the process of detoxification and prevent the resolution of symptoms associated with food allergy. The majority of my patients succeed in the detoxification process because they quickly feel so much better, motivating them to stick with the program. To prevent blood sugar swings, I suggest snacks between meals using nuts, seeds, nut butters (excluding peanut), or other proteins including chicken, turkey, and fish. Filtered water, vegetable juices, and herbal teas are the preferred beverages.

If needed, psyllium seed husks or flaxseed powder can be added to assist detoxification at the first sign of constipation. It is important to avoid hidden refined sugars including any food with sucrose, fructose, high-fructose corn syrup, dextrose, honey, or other sweeteners. Artificial flavorings and colorings in processed and packaged foods, sodas, and all caffeinated beverages must go!

In addition, all gluten-containing grains, including wheat, rye, barley, spelt, and kamut are not allowed. Steel-cut slow-cooking oatmeal is allowed. Substitutes are buckwheat (not related to wheat), rice, tapioca, millet, and amaranth.

Shellfish, meat, pork, cold cuts, and sausage are eliminated in the detoxification process because of the presence of chemicals added in processing, antibiotics and hormones (used in raising beef), and contaminants in shellfish. Allowed protein includes free range-fed chicken and turkey, fish other than farm raised (if possible), lamb, and wild game. Cow's milk dairy products including cheese, yogurt, milk, and ice cream are not used because of the frequency of allergic response to these foods. Eggs are eliminated for the same reason. Menus and recipes are in the appendix (section 2).

Table 1: Foods for Phase One

	Foods to Include	Foods to Exclude
Fruits	Unsweetened fresh, frozen, water-packed, or canned fruits; fruit juices (except orange)	Orange, orange juice
Vegetables	All fresh, raw, steamed, sautéed, juiced, or roasted vegetables	Corn, creamed vegetables
Starch	Rice, oats, millet, quinoa, amaranth, teff, tapioca, buckwheat	Wheat, corn, barley, spelt, kamut, rye; all gluten-containing products

Bread/Cereal	Products made from rice, oat, buckwheat, millet, potato flour, tapioca, arrowroot, amaranth, quinoa, teff	Products made from wheat, spelt, kamut, rye, barley; all gluten-containing products
Legumes (vegetable protein)	All beans, peas, and lentils (unless otherwise indicated)	Soybeans, tofu, tempeh, soy milk, other soy products
Nuts and Seeds	Almonds, cashews, walnuts, sesame (tahini), sunflower, pumpkin seeds; butters made from these nuts and seeds	Peanuts, peanut butter
Meat and Fish (animal protein)	All canned (water-packed), frozen, or fresh fish, chicken, turkey, wild game, lamb	Beef, pork, cold cuts, frankfurters, sausage, canned meats, eggs, shellfish
Dairy Products and Milk Substitutes	Milk substitutes such as rice milk, almond milk, oat milk, coconut milk, and other nut milks	Milk, cheese, cottage cheese, cream, yogurt, butter, ice cream, frozen yogurt, non-dairy creamers
Fats	Cold-expeller pressed olive, flaxseed, canola, grapeseed, sesame, walnut, pumpkin, or almond oils	Margarine, butter, shortening, processed and hydrogenated oils, mayonnaise, spreads, sunflower or safflower oil
Beverages	Filtered or distilled water, herbal tea, seltzer, or mineral water	Soda pop or soft drinks, alcoholic beverages, coffee, tea, other caffeinated beverages
Spices and Condiments	All spices unless otherwise indicated. For example, cinnamon, cumin, dill, garlic, ginger, carob, oregano, parsley, rosemary, tarragon, thyme, turmeric, vinegar	Chocolate, ketchup, mustard, relish, chutney, soy sauce, barbecue sauce, or other condiments

Sweeteners	Brown rice syrup, fruit sweetener, blackstrap molasses, stevia	White or brown refined sugar, honey, maple syrup, corn syrup, high fructose corn syrup, candy, desserts made with these sweeteners

(From Metagenics Ultraclear™ Patient Guide)

This phase of the Adaptation Diet accomplishes two important goals: avoidance of foods that are contaminated with chemicals including colorings, preservatives, additives, pesticide residues, hormones, industrial pollutants; and avoidance of common allergic foods. Through reduction in chemical exposure and food triggers of inflammation, the detoxification system can recover and become more efficient, reducing cortisol production. In the long run, this is the bottom line for healthy aging.

In my practice I often use a "medical food" protein powder that enhances the liver detoxification process. Use a powder that is a hypoallergenic rice-based protein that includes nutrients needed for the two phases of liver detoxification. (It is best if these products are used under medical supervision.) If this powder or a similar product is not used, it is possible to accomplish the same effect by adding the following supplements during the first five weeks of the diet. In addition, use protein-rich snacks between meals.

Table 2: Supplements for Phase One and Two

- A multivitamin and mineral not containing yeast, soy, wheat, sugar, or corn with at least 200 International Units of mixed tocopherols (vitamin E)
- Vitamin C (buffered with calcium and magnesium) 500–1000 milligrams (mg)
- N-acetylcysteine 100 mg
- Alpha lipoic acid 100 mg
- EPA/DHA fish oils 700 mg
- Bromelain enzymes (unless allergic to pineapple) twice daily between meals

At the end of three weeks on the detoxification diet, most people will notice improvement in fatigue, anxiety, moodiness, muscle and joint pain, headaches, and digestive problems and will lose between two and eight pounds. The weight loss is from water weight produced by inflammatory reactions to the foods that were eliminated. There are some people who will not notice much of a change during the detoxification phase, either in weight loss or symptom improvement. In those cases, if significant symptoms continue, additional medical evaluation is warranted.

The Food Allergy Challenge

Identifying foods that trigger inflammation and a wide range of symptoms is a major step along the path to adaptation and healthy aging. I could site hundreds of case histories demonstrating the impact food intolerance has on health.

Mary was a good example of the effect food allergy has on adaptation. Mary had chronic headaches, neck pain, and TMJ (temperomandibular joint disorder, a common problem of jaw pain and clicking when chewing that can be quite disabling). She had been to many specialists who devised mouth guards and treated her with pain medications and physical therapy. None of the therapies had made much difference despite many years of committed treatments. Mary knew that stress was a trigger, but despite her best efforts she had difficulty relaxing.

I put her on the Adaptation Diet and within ten days her pain had disappeared. During Phase Two of the diet, the food challenge, Mary reintroduced corn and found her pain return within two hours of eating corn on the cob and popcorn. Several days later she re-created her pain again after eating tomatoes and drinking tomato juice.

Once she adopted a diet eliminating corn and tomatoes and stayed with the anti-inflammatory maintenance phase of the Adaptation Diet, Mary continued to be pain free. If she strayed from her diet and had corn or tomato products, she had symptoms within the next few hours. She also noted an effect that I have seen many times after eliminating food allergens. She was more relaxed and handled stress more easily. This was not surprising because her allostatic load had been reduced, calming down her cortisol and epinephrine production. Most of my patients are able to reintroduce the allergic food in a rotation diet (see appendix section 4) within three to four months of elimination. Rarely does a food need to be eliminated indefinitely.

Phase Two: Weeks Four and Five

By the time Phase Two has been reached, the hard part is over. Generally after avoidance of an allergic food for three weeks, symptoms and allostatic load associated with that food have been reduced. Phase One of the diet has eliminated all the common food allergy triggers. By avoiding these foods, most people will have "unmasked," meaning that the next time they eat the food, if they are allergic to it, symptoms will be more noticeable and quicker to occur. This makes Phase Two of the diet so instructive in realizing the connection between foods and specific symptoms.

There is one caveat to the food challenge: anyone with asthma or a history of severe reactions to foods should not undertake the food challenge without medical supervision. Severe food reactions are typically limited to foods that trigger IgE antibodies (involved with immediate hypersensitivity and anaphylaxis) and include peanuts, Brazil and other nuts, shellfish, and strawberries.

The food challenge part of the diet requires good record keeping while carefully following the rules. Use only the forms of the food listed below to do the challenge. For example, wheat can only be tested using Shredded Wheat or matzo, not bread, since there are many other ingredients in a slice of bread. Symptoms generally occur within the first few hours; however they might be delayed as much as twenty-four hours. Reactions to these foods are generally mild and consist of headaches, fatigue, digestive upset, mood changes, poor concentration, or muscle and joint pain.

Use at least two portions of the challenge food with two different meals in addition to the foods from the Phase One diet. If symptoms occur, do not challenge another food until the symptoms resolve, usually within twenty-four hours. Record all symptoms in a diary so that you can review these at a later date if symptoms reoccur. Think of this exercise as empowering, not restricting. Many of my patients are upset to discover food allergies because it restricts their gustatory freedom. However, knowledge of food allergy provides control over symptoms and premature aging. For Mary, the trade-off of not eating corn in order to be free of her TMJ pain was a no-brainer.

The Food Challenge

The most common and significant food allergies are to wheat, corn, soy, dairy, beef, tomatoes, and yeast. The two-week period of Phase Two can be extended to test additional foods if needed. Don't deviate from the diet restrictions of Part One, especially avoiding sweets, coffee, and any fast foods. Starting with wheat on day one, each food to be challenged should be added in sizable portions to two consecutive meals. Observe symptoms over the subsequent twenty-four hours and keep a diary of foods introduced and symptoms. If there are no symptoms by the following day, a new food can be tested. As mentioned before, if symptoms occur, no new food should be introduced until they have cleared. If it is unclear whether there were significant symptoms, challenge the food again after waiting at least four days to retest. To hasten clearing of food allergy symptoms, drink at least 64 ounces of purified water, increase vitamin C intake to 2000 mg for a few days, and use Alka-Seltzer Gold (only Gold has the right bicarbonate mix) as directed. Wait to challenge the next food until symptoms have cleared. Below are the specifics on food challenge for the major allergic foods

- *Wheat*—Use Shredded Wheat, matzo, wheat crackers without yeast, wheat pasta, or pure wheat cereals. Do not use bread since it contains multiple ingredients. If there is no reaction to wheat, it can be kept in the diet but only in whole wheat or sprouted wheat forms.

- *Dairy*—Cow's milk (whole), plain unsweetened yogurt, and cottage cheese are recommended for challenging. Ice cream and aged cheeses (Swiss, cheddar, blue, etc.) are not to be used. Butter has no milk protein, so it is not used as a challenge food. If lactose intolerance is an issue, this challenge should be avoided. Digestive symptoms are common with dairy products in people that have not eaten them in a while. If dairy is tolerated in the food challenge, I recommend only the use of low-fat yogurts and kefirs to reduce the inflammatory response to the fats in dairy. Organic dairy products are strongly recommended to reduce the inflammatory fatty acids.

- *Corn*—Fresh corn on the cob, canned corn (not creamed), popcorn (plain without flavorings), or polenta (corn flour) can be used. Corn is one of the most common adulterants in prepared foods including corn syrup, cornstarch, high-fructose sweeteners, corn meal, and other ingredients. If symptoms from corn are identified in the food challenge, then reading labels is essential. Even if there is no allergy, avoidance of foods sweetened with corn syrup products leads to better blood sugar control and less cortisol production.

- *Beef*—Six to eight ounces of beef, preferably organically raised, is the best way to test for beef allergy. If there are no symptoms, most people should use only small portions of beef at most once a week because of the inflammatory fatty acids and saturated fats in beef. Organically raised beef is much better in terms of these fats.

- *Eggs*—Two or three eggs at a serving preferably boiled or poached is the best challenge. Eggs have enormous differences in fatty acid composition between organically fed and free-range birds. Only eggs from free-range and organically fed birds should be consumed. If eggs trigger symptoms in the food challenge, it is possible that chicken itself is an allergen and should be tested separately. If eggs are tolerated, they are best prepared by boiling or poaching, not breaking the yolk during cooking. Depending on a person's cholesterol levels, eggs can be eaten twice weekly.
- *Soy*—Challenge with plain soymilk, roasted soybeans, tofu, or tempeh. Do not use sweetened soymilk. With the tremendous increase in soy use during the past decade, I have seen many more soy allergies. If the test for soy is positive, read labels diligently to avoid the many products with soy as a filler or stabilizer.
- *Yeast*—Baker's yeast is a common allergen and can be tested by eating bread if wheat and dairy are not problematic. The other option is adding a package of nutritional yeast to water or juice. Yeast allergy is often seen with chronic digestive symptoms or recurrent respiratory infections.
- Other foods that can be tested include tomatoes, pork, sugar, coffee, black tea, potatoes, oranges, chocolate, peanuts (if no history of severe allergic reactions), and food colorings.

When Phase Two is completed, whether it takes two weeks or longer, the maintenance Phase Three of the Adaptation Diet is begun. All foods that tested positive need to be avoided for the next three months. At that point, these foods can be reintroduced one at a time. If no symptoms are noted, they can be used as often as twice a week for the subsequent three months. (See appendix section 4 for rotation diet example)

Food Allergy and Cortisol—A Key to Adaptation

Adaptation and reduction of allostatic load can only be achieved if the biochemical stress from food allergies and food intolerance is taken into account. Food allergy and intolerance is a major cause of maladaptation. Studies estimate that as many as one in every two Americans might have some level of food allergy or intolerance. Symptoms triggered by food allergy promote inflammation and changes in the hormonal system leading to an elevated cortisol burden. Most physicians never take into account the possibility that food intolerance can be contributing to a host of symptoms (see tables 3 and 4). Every day in my practice, patients report dramatic improvement in a host of symptoms from diet changes based on food allergy testing.

Table 3: Symptoms of Delayed Food Hypersensitivity

- Asthma and recurrent respiratory infections
- Nasal congestion and discharge
- Skin rash, eczema, hives
- Recurrent ear infections, fluid in ear, dizziness
- Recurrent yeast vaginitis
- All chronic digestive disorders—bloating, gas, heartburn, reflux, diarrhea, constipation, irritable bowel, and colitis
- Frequent urination, recurrent bladder infections, burning, bed wetting in children
- Fatigue and lethargy
- Depression, moodiness, and anxiety
- Headaches and migraine
- Joint pains, arthritis, unexplained muscle pain
- Hyperactivity and ADD, ADHD
- Cognitive dysfunction—poor concentration
- Eczema and hives
- Obesity and food cravings

Table 4: Signs of Food Allergy in Children

- Allergic shiners (dark circles under eyes)
- Allergic salute (rubbing the nose and eyes)
- Difficulty sitting still, restlessness
- Red earlobes
- Clearing throat excessively
- Nasal congestion
- Frequent vague stomach pains
- Impulsivity, distractibility

I have been guiding my patients on their diets since I started my practice in 1978. In 1980, I attended the training program presented by the Society for Clinical Ecology (now known as the American Academy of Environmental Medicine) at a retreat center in the Rocky Mountains outside of Fort Collins, Colorado. It was one of the most important professional decisions I ever made, dramatically changing the way I practiced medicine.

One of my good friends in medical school had spent a year with the founder of Clinical Ecology, Theron Randolph, MD. Randolph was a traditional allergist who discovered that foods, molds, and chemicals—including natural gas, phenol, benzene, and other common man-made products—were triggering a wide range of symptoms in his patients. (Other pioneers in the area of environmental medicine who broke ranks with their allergist colleagues in the 1930s and 1940s included Herbert Rinkel, Albert Rowe, and Arthur Coca.) Randolph painstakingly recorded detailed histories from his patients, identifying the culprits in problems such as fatigue, depression, arthritis, digestive problems, asthma, and other allergic symptoms. He hospitalized his most difficult patients in an environmental control unit where they had no exposure to common food allergies or chemicals that might cause problems. He then challenged his patients with foods that triggered their symptoms, discovering that many of these chronic complaints were caused by commonly eaten foods.

What amazed Randolph and revolutionized the field of food allergy was the wide range of symptoms caused by foods that had previously been unrecognized. Traditional allergy practice limited the scope of symptoms attributed to foods to only those mediated by IgE antibodies, including hives, eczema, allergic rhinitis, asthma, and acute diarrhea. (There are several types of antibodies that contribute to allergic responses. Traditional allergists concern themselves only with IgE, which causes histamine release. A different antibody, IgG, and cell-based responses are associated with delayed sensitivity to foods.) It became gospel that any other symptom could not be triggered by a food. The traditional allergists were wrong. In my own practice, the most common symptoms I find from foods are fatigue, tension, anxiety, insomnia, headaches, migraines, depression, joint pains, and digestive upsets (including heartburn, reflux, bloating and gas, constipation, and diarrhea). Even in patients without major medical issues, symptoms of maladaptation can be triggered by foods.

The controversy surrounding the notion that food allergies cause such widespread symptoms has to do with the difference between delayed and immediate reactions. Symptoms from immediate food reactions are mediated through histamine release and include hives, wheezing, swelling of the face or throat (anaphylaxis when severe), itching eyes or throat, and runny nose. It is obvious to people who suffer from this problem what foods triggered their reaction since it occurs within minutes of ingestion. These reactions are considered fixed food allergies that do not change or vary over a person's life. If you react to Brazil nuts with breathing problems or anaphylaxis as a child, this will probably continue even into adulthood and should be avoided. The most common foods for immediate sensitivity include peanuts, shellfish, Brazil and other nuts, and strawberries. Most of the time, these problems can be avoided by identifying the food trigger, reading labels, and asking at restaurants about ingredients.

Delayed food reactions, also called cyclic, can occur up to twenty-four hours after eating a food, though most commonly the response is within several hours. The symptoms are not as dramatic and sudden, often involving vague problems including fatigue, sore muscles, joint pain, headaches, mild depression, and a feeling of general unwellness. Though vague and often not severe, every time a food triggers symptoms, the body responds with increased cortisol and the attending allostatic load. This is why identifying food allergy and changing diets is so important in regaining adaptation.

Part of the difficulty in identifying food triggers for these symptoms is a phenomenon known as masking. When a food is eaten repetitively, even though it might cause an immunological or biochemical response, symptoms can be hidden or masked and not recognized. For example, fatigue, pain, depression, or other symptoms might be triggered by wheat, however if wheat is eaten every day, a masked state occurs and no cause and effect will be noticed. However, if there is a period of avoidance, such as Phase One of the diet, unmasking will occur, and when the food is reintroduced, symptoms will be more obvious.

John, a patient who is wheat intolerant (he did not know it at the time), traveled to China on vacation, where at that time no wheat products were available. He felt more energetic and less achy or moody during the trip, though he assumed it was because of the vacation and the incredible experience of touring China. When John returned and resumed his normal eating habits, including wheat cereal in the morning and sandwiches daily, the fatigue and muscle aches returned with a vengeance. He never thought that his diet was the culprit.

When he relayed this story to me, I asked him to stop eating wheat for a week and then reintroduce it. The same sequence happened: his fatigue and muscle aches improved when he stopped eating wheat and returned once he ate wheat again. We then skin tested John for food allergy to confirm the sensitivity to wheat. John had unmasked his wheat allergy during his trip and the test period. By doing this, he moved from an adapted state in which there was a hidden price to pay for the wheat intolerance (fatigue and muscle aches) to a preadapted state where the symptoms are gone but when exposed the reaction to an allergic food will be stronger. This technique of unmasking is the reason that a simple home testing approach (avoidance and challenge), which is Phase Two of the Adaptation Diet, helps to identify food offenders.

When a person eats a food to which they are intolerant (let's take corn for example), the protein in the corn, after digestion in the gut and absorption through the small intestine wall into the bloodstream, triggers a response in the immune system that causes joint pain (or any one of many other symptoms) through release of immune hormones including lymphokines, cytokines, interferons, and histamine. The immune cells in the gut, which comprises nearly half of the entire immune system, can also react to the allergen, leading to inflammation and digestive problems. Symptoms might be delayed up to twenty-four hours (though most commonly they would be seen within six hours), making the connection to corn as the culprit very difficult. If corn was repeatedly eaten, a more continual joint pain might ensue, usually without the characteristics of serious arthritis like rheumatoid or osteoarthritis. (Findings common for inflammatory arthritis such as redness, swelling, and heat are not typically seen with food reactions.)

Using joint pain triggered by corn as an example, let's see how most physicians would approach this problem. A battery of blood tests and X-rays would be ordered to identify the type of arthritis. Treatment with anti-inflammatory medications would probably follow. In this situation, lab tests would be normal. While initially a response to medications might be favorable, in the long run ironically these medications can actually intensify food allergy.

Most nonsteroidal anti-inflammatory (NSAIDs) medications work by preventing the enzymes, COX-1 and COX-2 from triggering leukotrienes that cause inflammation. Unfortunately, this enzyme is also used by the digestive tract to ensure membrane integrity (the reason one side effect of these drugs is stomach ulcers). Another little-known side effect of these medications is an increase in intestinal permeability that allows the absorption of larger-than-normal proteins from the digestion of foods. These proteins are interpreted by the immune system as foreign substances, which can lead to more antibody production by the immune system and intensify food allergy. Therefore, treating joint pain triggered by corn with ibuprofen (or other anti-inflammatory medication) will work for a time, but eventually it will make the problem worse. The solution is to recognize the effect food can have on chronic symptoms and change the diet.

Not surprisingly, the most common foods that trigger delayed food allergy are the ones most Americans eat the most: milk, cheese, wheat, yeast, soy, corn, eggs, sugar, beef, and tomatoes. When I put my patients on an allergy free diet that avoids the major allergens and also takes out all processed foods, sugar, and desserts, remarkable changes occur in most of their main complaints. Headaches, fatigue, joint pain, and digestive problems frequently improve within weeks. To identify the food triggers after an elimination diet, reintroduction of each food one at a time often re-creates a person's symptoms. For people with medical problems or multiple allergies, consulting a physician who specializes in food allergies, such as members of the American Academy of Environmental Medicine, is the best approach.

How is one to suspect food allergy? Here are some hints. A history of any respiratory allergy including hay fever, asthma, nasal congestion, or itching nose, eyes, or throat makes food allergy likely. Itching in the ear canal, rectal itching, and itching between the shoulder blades also can indicate food allergy. Any family history of allergy increases the likelihood of food intolerance. A childhood history of colic, chronic digestive problems, bedwetting, carsickness, recurrent ear infections, tonsillitis, and frequent colds is suspicious. Frequent respiratory or urinary infections, chronic digestive complaints including gas, bloating, constipation, diarrhea, and skin rashes are usually a sign of food allergy in an adult. Unexplained fatigue, mood changes, and depression can all be caused by food allergy. Probably the most common complaints from my food-allergic patients are fatigue, aches and pains, and the inability to lose weight.

Many of my patients ask why they have developed food allergies. People who have strong genetic predispositions for allergies often have sensitivities to pollens, molds, and dust as well as foods. They typically have respiratory symptoms such as hay fever and asthma. However, the majority of food-intolerant patients have developed this problem over time rather than through a strong genetic component. The digestive tract is often the culprit. As I mentioned earlier, the use of anti-inflammatory medications impacts the integrity of the gut wall leading to a leaky gut, which in turn causes absorption of larger molecules from food and an allergic response.

Antibiotics also play a major role in initiating food allergy by reducing the number of protective bacterial organisms in the digestive tract. This leads to overgrowth of unwanted bacteria and yeast (*Candida albicans*) or susceptibility to parasitic organisms. With fewer lactic- acid-forming bacteria, the gut wall is susceptible to leaky gut and food allergy. In addition, abnormal organisms in the gut trigger a brisk immune response that can lead to excessive reactivity to foods. *Candida albicans* is especially problematic because it adheres to the gut wall and directly contributes to a leaky gut.

Acid-blocking medications (Zantac, Prilosec, Tagamet to name a few) alter the digestive process by reducing stomach acid secretion. (These are important drugs when needed to treat gastritis, gastric reflux, or ulcers but are widely overused by physicians and the public.) With less stomach acid comes reduced pancreatic enzyme secretion, leading to poor digestion of proteins and absorption of substances triggering allergy. These drugs also contribute to nutritional deficiencies (B12, zinc, and other minerals) that affect the immune system as well.

Poor nutritional habits lead to greater food allergy incidence through continual exposure to the same foods, fast foods, sugars, and unhealthy oils and fats. The typical American diet, rich in omega 6 fats and simple sugars and lacking omega 3 fats and complex carbohydrates, impacts the digestive process by encouraging abnormal bacteria growth in the gut while not providing the nutrients needed for the health of the gut wall cells, the mucocytes. Poor nutrition can lead to greater likelihood of viral illness that can at times trigger a food allergy problem.

The change in food composition of the American diet also plays a role. The number of food additives has skyrocketed over the past thirty years, leading to recurrent exposure to chemicals in foods. Foods containing preservatives, conditioners, and artificial colorings and flavorings, and foods that are contaminated with antibiotics from animal feed and pesticides add to the impact on the immune system in the digestive tract. Other behaviors such as early weaning and premature introduction of solid foods to infants and the repetitive nature of most diets have been suggested to increase food intolerances.

Not only do food allergies increase the allostatic load and cortisol burden, food allergies themselves are the result of long-term stress. Allostasis and high cortisol levels inhibit the normal immune response in the gut, leading to more infections. High cortisol also raises stomach acid production, leading to more use of acid-blocking drugs, and furthering malabsorption. Chronic stress and allostastic load will eventually change the immune response, leading to more allergies. Managing food allergies is a major part of the dietary control of cortisol and regaining adaptation.

Studies of the most common chronic symptoms associated with food allergies and intolerance have led to many useful findings in designing a diet to improve adaptation and well-being. In a study of migraine patients reported by Ellen Grant in the *Lancet*, 85 percent became headache free after going on an elimination diet. The most common food triggers were as follows:

- Wheat—78 percent
- Orange—65 percent
- Eggs—45 percent
- Tea and coffee—40 percent each
- Chocolate and milk—37 percent each
- Beef—35 percent
- Corn, cane sugar, and yeast—33 percent each

In children with migraines in another study, seventy-eight of eighty-eight became symptom free during a strict elimination diet. When foods were reintroduced, the most common that triggered reactions were, in order of frequency: milk, eggs, chocolate, orange, wheat, benzoic acid, cheese, tomato, fish, pork, beef, corn, and soy. Many other studies have confirmed the importance of food allergy in migraine as well as tension headaches.

Headaches are easier to study than many other symptoms because they are episodic. However, digestive problems such as irritable bowel syndrome, inflammatory bowel disease, gall bladder symptoms, gastritis, and other problems have been shown definitively to have a link with food allergy. Irritable bowel syndrome is a chronic condition with alternating diarrhea, constipation, cramps, and mucous in the stool. It is not progressive and involves no pathological changes in the gut wall, though many patients have symptoms that greatly impact their well-being. I have found food intolerance and allergy to be a major component in many of my IBS patients. In a study with double-blind feeding challenges, two thirds of the patients showed increased levels of prostaglandins in their stool, indicating an inflammatory reaction to the foods. The most common foods in order of reactivity for IBS patients were wheat, corn, dairy, coffee, tea, and oranges.

Other studies have shown that elimination diets help over half the people with IBS. In a study of 189 patients by Nanda (*Gut* 1989), most reacted to between two and five foods, with the most common as follows: dairy 40 percent, onions 35 percent, wheat 29 percent, chocolate 27 percent, coffee 24 percent, eggs 23 percent, oranges 18 percent, tea 17 percent, and potatoes 15 percent. Of 73 patients who avoided their symptom-provoking foods, 72 remained well for longer than a year.

Children with attention deficit hyperactivity disorder (ADHD) often have food allergies as a trigger for their behavioral and cognitive symptoms. There is a great deal of controversy over the effect that diet and especially food colorings and additives have on these children. However, in a recent study, nineteen out of twenty-six children placed on an elimination diet improved. Children with allergy histories such as eczema or hay fever were more likely to be reactive to the food challenge. The most common provoking agents were corn, wheat, milk, soy, food color, and oranges. My experience confirms the importance of evaluating food allergies in these children especially if they have a respiratory allergy history or a family history of allergies. Even in adults with ADD, food allergies play a major role.

Other areas that research has found food allergy to be a significant trigger for symptoms include bed wetting in children, asthma, allergic rhinitis, hives, ear infections, and arthritis. Joint and muscle pain are symptoms that I have found to be commonly triggered by food allergy. My patients with poorly defined muscle and joint pain, often diagnosed with fibromyalgia, myofascial pain, sero-negative arthritis, arthralgia, and myalgia, frequently improve by identifying and eliminating food allergies. Even in rheumatoid arthritis, food allergies can contribute to symptoms.

Table 5: Conditions Found to Have a Food Allergy Component

- Irritable bowel syndrome
- Gall bladder disease
- Inflammatory bowel disease
- Allergic rhinitis
- Asthma
- Eczema
- ADHD, ADD in children and adults
- Rheumatoid arthritis
- Fibromyalgia, myofascial pain
- Arthralgia and myalgia
- Bed wetting in children
- Migraine and tension headaches
- Chronic fatigue

The bottom line is that any patient with chronic symptoms that are not easily treated with medical therapy and cannot be easily explained deserves to be evaluated for food allergies by a well-trained physician. Even if the problems are less serious but involve reduced quality of life and well-being, changes in diet and avoidance of food triggers as described in the Adaptation Diet will reduce allostatic load and improve adaptation.

Rotary Diversified Diet—A Solution for Multiple Food Allergies

The rotation diet has been a core approach in managing food allergies. There are many benefits to the rotation diet not the least of which is unmasking the symptoms caused by food allergy. The original idea of a four-day rotation comes from studying gut transit times, or how long a food takes to completely leave the body. While food remnants remain in the gut, it is possible that the immune system continues to react to the food through production of antibodies or cell-based immune responses. It appears that for most people with a typical fiber intake, four days is the time it takes to clear a food completely from the digestive tract.

Based on this information the four-day rotation became the standard of managing food allergies. Additionally, since foods of the same family might cause similar allergic responses, rotating through food families is also recommended. Using chicken as an example, if this was part of Monday's food intake, it should not be eaten again until Friday. In addition, other foods of the same family, like eggs, should also be rotated on those days. The benefit beyond unmasking reactions to foods is to reduce the likelihood of creating additional allergic reactions to tolerated foods. The rotation diet supports the process of desensitization and tolerance, reducing allostatic load.

For most people, rotation of the whole diet is not needed unless food allergy is a major problem. Foods that are symptom triggers discovered through the challenge part of the Adaptation Diet require avoidance for three to four months. This usually brings back tolerance, but if symptoms still occur when reintroducing the food, then a four-day rotation diet makes sense. The bottom line is that the more variety in one's diet, the less likely one is to develop a food allergy.

For tens of thousands of generations, humans have been hunter-gatherers, picking berries and fruits and fishing and hunting game for food. There was no repetitive exposure to foods, since you ate what was available and then moved on to the next food source. Until the cultivation of grains and the rise of cities, this was the diet of *homo sapiens*. Compare that to how we eat now. Most people eat the same limited number of foods every day. Seasonal availability is often overcome by transporting foods from other continents so that the same meals can be consumed regardless of season or time of year.

The repetitive nature of our diets is one of the causes of the epidemic of food allergy. The rotation diet, encouraging the maximum variety of food, can modulate this problem and prevent additional allergies and intolerance. Even incorporating just some of these concepts improves adaptation. For many people, a strict four-day rotation diet is not necessary. However, knowledge of food families as well as awareness of the need for variety will encourage greater adaptation, lower allostatic load, and improved cortisol control.

The appendix (section 4) contains lists of food families, examples of four-day rotation diets, and suggested rotations. This can be incorporated into the maintenance Adaptation Diet by rotating foods as possible. If there is evidence of multiple food allergies on the food challenge and symptoms that point to other food allergies, the four-day rotation of the Adaptation Diet is critical. With any chronic medical condition, the rotation diet should be supervised by a physician with training in environmental medicine. For those people who do not have any evidence of food allergy, simply trying to get the greatest variety possible in the diet will suffice.

Chapter Five

Phase Three of the Adaptation Diet: Control Inflammation and Maintain Healthy Cortisol Levels throughout Life

Maintaining adaptation in the diet is a major contributor to balanced cortisol levels and healthy aging. Completing Phase One of the Adaptation Diet improves the detoxification pathways and removes offending foods. Phase Two identifies food intolerance and allergy. Phase Three builds on the benefits of detoxification and identification of food allergies to create a dietary program that controls cortisol, helps achieve normal body weight, and supports healthy aging.

The long-term goal of the Adaptation Diet is the reduction of allostatic load from poor dietary habits that trigger inflammation, allergies, insulin resistance, and hypoglycemia. The diet is rich in foods that normalize cortisol response—high-fiber beans, adequate amounts of low-fat protein, flaxseeds, omega 3 fats from fish and nuts, carotenoids and flavonoids from vegetables and fruit, and sulfides for detoxification from garlic, onions, and cruciferous vegetables.

The Adaptation Diet is a modern version of the Mediterranean diet that has been proven to reduce overall mortality, especially heart disease and cancer. The Adaptation Diet is not really a diet, but a life-long pattern of consuming health-enhancing foods. At every meal, the goal is to seek out the foods that improve adaptation and healthy aging and avoid those that induce inflammation, blood sugar problems, and allergic reactions. There is no doubt that healthy aging depends on eating correctly.

Fats and Adaptation

The typical American diet promotes inflammation through the use of a higher percentage of animal foods and processed foods containing omega-6 fats (linoleic acid) and trans fats. One hundred years ago (and currently in most traditional diets worldwide), the ratio of omega 6 to omega 3 fats was between 2:1 and 4:1. Today, in the average American diet, the ratio is closer to 25:1, dramatically increasing inflammation in every organ of the body. In addition, the poisonous trans fats introduced by the food industry over the past thirty years directly increase free radical production, damaging cell membranes and triggering additional inflammation.

The fats that are so crucial to adaptation are more correctly termed essential fatty acids (EFA). These nutrients are not made in the body; therefore, diet or supplements are needed to obtain these critical substances. EFAs are incorporated into cell membranes throughout the body, especially in the brain and nervous system. They are needed for the transport of nutrients, chemical messengers, hormones, and neurotransmitters into cells, leading to normal cell function. The integrity of the cell membrane and organelles inside the cell is dependent on normal fatty acids.

Essential fatty acids are important in energy production, oxygen transport, cell-to-cell communication, and the myelination of neurons in the central nervous system. They are the building blocks of the eicosanoid hormones and the prostaglandins, which are key regulators of inflammation in the body. Any change in the dietary intake of fats has a profound effect on cell membranes, cell function, and levels of inflammatory hormones. It's no wonder that so many studies have confirmed the importance of eating the right fats to maintain health.

One example of the impact of using unhealthy fats is a recent study on ulcerative colitis, a severe inflammatory bowel disease. Nearly a third of ulcerative colitis cases may be associated with high dietary levels of linoleic acid, according to a study by A.R. Hart published in July 2009 in *Gut*. Linoleic acid is an omega-6 polyunsaturated fatty acid found in red meat and some cooking oils and margarine.

Over 200,000 subjects in five European countries submitted food-frequency questionnaires at the start of the study, and incident cases of ulcerative colitis were identified from disease registries, follow-up questionnaires, and hospital and pathology databases. After a median follow-up of four years, those with the highest quartile of linoleic acid intake showed a 2.5-fold increased risk for ulcerative colitis relative to the lowest quartile.

There are several types of fatty acids found in foods. Fats from animal products including meat and dairy contain saturated fats and arachidonic acid, an omega 6 fatty acid that increases levels of pro-inflammatory prostaglandin hormones. Monounsaturated fats (also called omega 9) are neutral and stable fats that are generally anti-inflammatory. Polyunsaturated fats include both omega 6 and omega 3 fatty acids. Most omega 6 fatty acids are pro-inflammatory, including those found in corn oil, safflower oil, soybean oil, peanut oil, and cottonseed oil. However, some omega 6 oils are beneficial and can be used as supplements, including those found in primrose oil, borage and black currant seed oils. (They contain gamma linoleic acid, a healthy EFA.) Omega 3 fatty acids, found in cold-water fish and flaxseeds, support the anti-inflammatory prostaglandin hormones and are the most beneficial in controlling inflammation.

Trans fats, a synthetic chemical used to make liquid fats solid (as in margarine), are also called hydrogenated or partially hydrogenated oils. Trans is the mirror image of the normal fatty acid configuration, called cis. When these oils are incorporated into cell membranes, they become stiff and reduce their membrane transport function. This leads to cell dysfunction and has been associated with increased risk for heart disease and increased inflammation. Unfortunately, trans fats are found in many processed foods, including chips, cookies, soups, pastries, French fries, margarine, and fast foods. Recently, the food industry has finally accepted the decades-old research that proved these fats are dangerous and has begun removing them from a number of products.

(The current USDA Food Guide Pyramid does not make the distinction between healthy fats like monounsaturated oils and unhealthy fats like saturated, found mostly in red meats and tropical oils, and trans fats found mostly in margarines, snack foods, processed peanut butter, and commercial baked goods.)

A major step in reducing inflammation and controlling cortisol is choosing the right fats—omega 3 fats from cold-water fish: wild salmon, sardines, herring, low-mercury tuna, as well as vegetable sources: flaxseeds, walnuts, pepitas, and dark green leafy vegetables. Monounsaturated fats from almonds, avocado, olive oil, grapeseed oil, and canola oil should be the main fats in the diet. In addition, strictly avoid trans fats. Also reduce the use of polyunsaturated omega 6 fats found in corn oil, safflower oil, soybean oil, and other partially hydrogenated oils. Reducing the intake of saturated fats from beef, whole dairy products, and egg yolks also decreases the inflammatory response.

The Mediterranean Experience

Just as important as avoidance of pro-inflammatory foods is the inclusion of foods that are anti-inflammatory. The Mediterranean diets found in Greece and Italy, shown to reduce markers of inflammation and thereby lead to less heart disease, cancer, diabetes, obesity and other aging phenomena, are templates for the construction of the Adaptation Diet. The characteristics of these diets are the following:

- Low-glycemic-index carbohydrates such as whole grains, fruits, and vegetable in large amounts
- Minimal snacking between meals and no fast foods
- Moderate consumption of red wine (5 ounces per day)
- Olive oil as the principal fat, with significant amounts of fish, nuts, and seeds and a balanced omega 6 to 3 ratio
- Significant intake of fish, especially salmon and small fish like sardines rich in EPA-DHA fatty acids
- Little saturated fats from butter, cream, full-fat dairy, or red meats
- Protein primarily as beans and lentils with moderate amounts of fish and poultry
- Dairy consumed as low-fat yogurt, kefir, or cheese
- Fat consumption is 25–35 percent of calories, with saturated fat less than 8 percent
- Desserts are fruits, often fresh
- Use of local produce, fish, and poultry with minimal importation from distant sources
- Slow food approach, eating leisurely meals in a social setting with family and friends

In a study of cortisol levels and hypothalamic-pituitary-adrenal (HPA) activity in women in the Mediterranean area, a disturbed HPA axis was associated with abdominal fat distribution and a higher content of fat and saturated fatty acids in the diet. Women who chose a dietary pattern closer to the Mediterranean diet, with high monounsaturated fatty acid intake, showed lower levels of HPA axis disturbance.

The Mediterranean diet protects against obesity and diabetes through reducing inflammation and cortisol elevation. It includes consumption of significant amounts of vegetables and fruits and using olive oil as the principal fat. Both epidemiological and interventional studies have revealed a protective effect of the Mediterranean diet against mild chronic inflammation and its metabolic complications. Mounting evidence suggests that Mediterranean diets could serve as an anti-inflammatory dietary pattern, which could help in fighting diseases that are related to chronic inflammation, including visceral obesity, heart disease, Type 2 diabetes, and the metabolic syndrome. There is also a lower incidence of several types of cancer with these dietary practices.

Dietary patterns close to the Mediterranean diet, rich in fruit and vegetables and high in monounsaturated fats, are negatively associated with features of the metabolic syndrome. The metabolic syndrome, also called syndrome X, includes high blood pressure, insulin resistance, truncal obesity, high triglycerides and blood sugar, and low HDL cholesterol. It is a major risk factor for heart disease and diabetes. Some recent studies, including one done by Balbio in Spain, have demonstrated a 25 percent net reduction in the prevalence of metabolic syndrome following lifestyle changes mainly based on nutritional recommendations.

Olive oil is also an integral ingredient of the Mediterranean diet, and accumulating evidence suggests that it may have health benefits that include reduction of risk factors of coronary heart disease, prevention of several varieties of cancers, and modification of immune and inflammatory responses. Olive oil appears to be an example of a functional food, with varied components that may contribute to its overall therapeutic characteristics. Olive oil is known for its high levels of monounsaturated fatty acids and is also a good source of phytochemicals including polyphenolic compounds, squalene, and alpha tocopherol (vitamin E). A unique characteristic of olive oil is its enrichment in oleuropein, a member of the secoiridoid family, which functions as a hydrophilic phenolic antioxidant.

Inhabitants of the Greek island of Crete are 20 percent less likely to die from coronary artery disease and have one-third the cancer rate of Americans. A study comparing foods that are typically found in a Greek diet to what is often consumed in the United States shows the following:

- Greeks ate much less red meat and used many more plant-based foods, averaging nine servings a day of antioxidant-rich vegetables.
- Greeks ate cold-water fish several times a week—another heart-healthy investment since fish contain omega-3 oils that not only reduce heart disease risk but also boost immune system functioning.
- The Greek diet contains little of the two kinds of fats known to raise blood cholesterol levels: saturated fat and trans fat.

Sugar, Carbohydrates, Metabolic Syndrome, and Adaptation

In the 1980s, under the leadership of the FDA and cardiologists nationwide, Americans were given an ultimatum: reduce your fat intake or die. All fats were bad, and little was made of the difference in fatty acids as previously discussed. Unfortunately, this fat-avoidance craze has actually resulted in even more obesity, more heart disease, and more diabetes. Over the past twenty years as low fat processed foods have flooded the grocery store, Americans have reached the highest percentage of obesity ever seen. The reason is that in most processed foods that are low fat, refined sugar products have been used to replace the fat. This leads to higher insulin levels and eventually insulin resistance. In fact, fat in food decreases overall caloric intake by leading to faster satiety and lower insulin response, leading to improved weight management. The reality is that research has shown that incorporating the right dietary fats (no more than 30 percent of daily calories) will lead to better weight management and less inflammation.

If the makers of nutrition policy had paid attention to an event that occurred as a result of the Cold War, possibly the fat-avoidance craze would have never happened. In the 1950s, the United States built the Distant Early Warning radar system in the Arctic regions of the United States and Canada. The construction was done in native Eskimo areas. At that time, there was essentially no heart disease or diabetes in these Native Americans, despite the fact that their diet had a huge percentage of calories from fat. They ate seal blubber and other animal fats. But they also ate no fast food and little sugar.

As "civilization" descended on these people and they adopted the sugar-rich, fast-food habits of most Americans, the incidence of heart disease, diabetes, and obesity skyrocketed. It wasn't the fats that caused these problems. It was the sugar and processed carbohydrates that were to blame. This taught me and others who were knowledgeable about nutrition that the low fat craze that started in the 1980s, ignoring the science such as the Eskimo studies, was bound to be a disaster.

These studies and many others have emphasized the need to restrict simple and refined carbohydrates and sugars to avoid blood sugar problems, which can lead to insulin resistance and more inflammation. Insulin, a hormone made in the pancreas, brings sugar from the bloodstream into the cell for energy production. As noted earlier, in insulin resistance cell-membrane receptors become inefficient at responding to the signal from insulin to produce the changes needed to absorb glucose into the cell. This leads to higher and higher levels of insulin and blood sugar. Insulin resistance is often the result of decades of poor dietary habits leading to abdominal obesity. Insulin resistance affects up to one third of the population and greatly increases the risk for diabetes, heart disease, cancer, and high blood pressure. Elevated insulin leads to more inflammation and higher cortisol levels.

Insulin receptors on the cell surface can be affected by hormones and chemical messengers made by adipocytes, the fat cells that are found in visceral or abdominal fat. Increased visceral fat increases inflammation through production of adipocytokines. They include TNF alpha and IL-6, which prevent insulin receptors from working well, increasing the risk for metabolic syndrome, diabetes, inflammation, and elevated cortisol levels.

The sequence of this all-too-common cycle of events starts with increased abdominal fat from using simple sugars and refined carbohydrates. For example, in one study, consumption of soft drinks was measured in middle-aged adults over a four-year period. Consumption of more than one soft drink per day increased the odds of developing metabolic syndrome and insulin resistance. After a period of time, and with weight gain of as little as nine pounds of visceral fat, insulin resistance can occur. Elevated insulin further increases abdominal obesity through mobilization of free fatty acids and movement of glucose into fat cells to store as extra calories. As the abdominal girth grows, these changes accelerate and increase the inflammatory state, leading to more insulin resistance at the cell membranes.

Increased free fatty acids from inflammatory chemicals made by fat cells (adipocytokines), like TNF alpha, increases triglycerides, insulin, and apolipoprotein B, leading to elevated cortisol and a marked increased risk of heart disease. Increased C-reactive protein and lower adiponectin, an anti-inflammatory adipocytokines that sensitizes cell-membrane insulin receptors, further worsens insulin resistance in obese people. Increased belly fat also leads to higher levels of resisten, a hormone that increases insulin resistance. These changes are the underlying events that lead to metabolic syndrome.

Metabolic syndrome is defined as having three of the following risk factors: increased waist girth—men above forty inches, women above thirty-five inches; blood sugar above 100 mg/dl; blood pressure above 130/85; triglycerides above 150. Here is where the story comes back to allostatic load and cortisol as a major component of these epidemic changes.

Many characteristics of metabolic syndrome are similar to Cushing's disease, a condition which is caused by either a pituitary or adrenal tumor secreting massive amounts of cortisol. The hallmark of Cushing's is visceral abdominal obesity, fatigue, mood changes, and marked increased risk for diabetes and heart disease. This has led several researchers to propose that the key hormonal change in the development of metabolic syndrome is not just insulin resistance, but continued elevation of cortisol production.

In a study by Vogelzangs (*American Journal of Geriatric Psychiatry*, 2009), of 1200 depressed older persons, those with higher levels of free cortisol showed higher odds of developing metabolic syndrome. Especially in women, depressive symptoms were associated with elevated afternoon and evening cortisol levels. In a review of the research from the past twenty years, the authors concluded that metabolic syndrome is associated with a state of "functional hypercortisolism" leading to increased fat deposition around the abdominal organs. In addition, the adipose tissue itself creates a huge amount of cortisol through the 11 beta-HSD1 enzyme system, which converts inactive cortisone to active cortisol, contributing to metabolic syndrome. The amount of cortisol produced by visceral fat is actually greater than what the adrenal gland produces in obese individuals, contributing to the biochemical chaos of the overweight state. Another study showed that once a person is obese, the normal feedback mechanism that shuts down cortisol production is impaired, contributing to this vicious cycle.

Signs of Metabolic Syndrome and Markers of Obesity

- Elevated blood pressure above 130/85
- Increased waist size: men, forty inches; women, thirty-five inches
- Blood glucose above 100 fasting
- Triglycerides above 150
- HDL less than 40 in men and 50 in women
- Elevated waist to hip ratio: greater than 1 in men and 0.8 in women
- Triglyceride to HDL ratio greater than 3
- Body mass index over 30
- Elevated GGT liver enzyme

Elevated levels of insulin have also been associated with high blood pressure as well as increased growth-factor production, leading to a higher incidence of cancers. All of this further impacts the level of cortisol, which is produced to counterbalance many of the effects of insulin, leading to even more damage from allostatic load. The key to reducing allostatic load and controlling cortisol excess and the risks for chronic disease is to reduce the amount of processed carbohydrates in the diet.

In addition, refined sugar and grains lead to a rapid spike in blood glucose and increased oxidant stress, leading to inflammation in just a few hours. The body's response is to produce more cortisol to reduce inflammation. Foods that cause a slower and more gradual and prolonged elevation of glucose do not cause the same inflammatory cascade and high cortisol levels. Several studies have shown that low-glycemic-carbohydrate based diets are more effective than low fat diets in treating obesity, metabolic syndrome, heart disease, and diabetes.

This is why the glycemic index is helpful in choosing what to eat. The glycemic index (GI) is a ranking of foods based on their potential to raise blood glucose. It compares the levels of blood sugar elevation after eating a portion of food and ranks them relative to glucose levels after either straight glucose ingestion or white bread. Low glycemic foods have a glycemic index below 55; high is above 70. For example, some candy bars have an index as high as 101, and corn flakes are 72, while an apple is 38, lentils are 29, and string beans are 32. In general, anything that is not whole and fresh probably has a high glycemic index.

However, some nutritious foods are listed as high GI although they really do not impact insulin production. For example watermelon and carrots have high GI marks though they do not create a negative impact on insulin sensitivity. The impact a food will have on blood sugar levels depends on many other factors, for instance: ripeness of a food, cooking time, fiber and fat content, time of day, blood insulin levels, and recent activity. Therefore, this index is not to be used in isolation. The total amount of carbohydrate, amount and type of fat, fiber and salt content, as well as the caloric value of a food are also very important. Another set of data, the glycemic load, has been developed to take into account all of these factors. The appendix (section 1) contains a table identifying glycemic index for some commonly used foods. The Internet has multiple sites to research glycemic load information.

Examples of High Glycemic Index Carbohydrates

Refined flour products including white bread, bagels
Frozen yogurt
Orange juice
Macaroni and cheese
Crackers
Candy
Cookies and all other desserts
Juice drinks with added sugar
White potatoes
Chips (corn and potato)
Most breakfast cereals
Sweetened soda

Selected Low Glycemic Index Carbohydrates

All-Bran cereal
Peaches, plums
Cherries
Barley
Grapefruit
Legumes (lentils, beans, peanuts)
Nuts (almonds, walnuts, soy nuts)
Oatmeal (steel cut, slow cook and unsweetened)

Green peas
Tomatoes
Unsweetened plain yogurt

Avoiding high-glycemic index food will reduce the likelihood of insulin resistance and metabolic syndrome. Low-glycemic diets have many benefits, including fewer food cravings, fewer calories consumed, and decreasing weight gain. In one study, those on a low-glycemic diet reported less hunger and showed lower serum triglycerides, blood pressure, and insulin resistance than higher glycemic diets. Higher beneficial HDL cholesterol was also noted.

The Adaptation Diet emphasizes the use of low GI vegetables, fruits, grains, proteins, and fats. The percentage of calories from the three major food groups should be as follows—mostly low-glycemic carbohydrates including predominately vegetables, legumes, and fruits and limited grains: 40–50 percent; protein from vegetarian and some animal sources: 30–40 percent; and fat from healthy oils, nuts, seeds, and fish: 20 percent. Carbohydrates including vegetables, legumes, and fruits are nature's powerhouse of adaptation containing thousands of beneficial phytonutrients including flavonoids, carotenoids, vitamins, minerals, and fiber.

Phytonutrients protect cell membranes, prevent damage to the cell nucleus, are required for detoxification by the liver and other organs, and help with normal cell-to-cell communication. They are the premier antioxidants, preventing inflammation and allostatic load and reducing the need for cortisol every time they are eaten. Numerous studies comparing American diets to Asian or other diets where there are much lower rates of cancer and heart disease show that one of the main differences is the lower level of phytonutrients in the American diet.

Protein sources should be carefully chosen as well. The best sources of protein as described in the Mediterranean diet include a balance between vegetarian sources such as legumes (beans), nuts, and seeds and fresh organic animal sources including fish and fowl, and if tolerated, low-fat unsweetened dairy (best as cultured foods such as yogurts and kefir). Protein is needed for every cell and organ in the body to maintain healthy function. It is the basis of muscle, skin, connective tissue, hormones, and all body proteins essential for life. Inadequate intake of protein leads to a breaking down of muscles and other vital organs and tissues to compensate. Weight management and normalizing blood glucose and insulin is best accomplished by eating protein at every meal and snack.

When to Eat

Another important point is not just what is eaten but when. As every mother would say, breakfast is the most important meal. Here is the reason. The circadian rhythm for cortisol appears to be deeply set in every person's brain. Cortisol levels peak at 8 a.m., preparing one for the challenges of the day. Cortisol gradually comes down during the course of the day, until it reaches a low point at midnight. Production is gradually ramped up during sleep, again peaking at 8 a.m.

One of the major effects of cortisol is raising blood sugar for brain function. Glucose is the fuel that is used by brain neurons to produce energy. In the morning, cortisol induces gluconeogenisis by converting protein (specific amino acids) into glucose and releasing glycogen from stores in muscle and the liver. Breakdown of muscle protein to satisfy the brain's need for glucose is one aspect of catabolism, an important, though potentially destructive function of cortisol.

To counteract the catabolic effects of cortisol, breakfast should contain high-quality protein to provide energy for the brain and stop breakdown of native tissue. The typical American breakfast of high-glycemic load, low-protein cereals, is exactly the opposite of what is needed at that time of day. Add a glass of orange juice, or worse, a juice drink that is loaded with added sugar, and a low fiber bread or muffin, and you have the makings of a veritable cortisol festival leading to additional catabolic effects including muscle loss and detrimental changes in body composition.

One other consequence of inadequate protein at breakfast is fluctuating blood glucose later in the day leading to hypoglycemia, another trigger for cortisol release. In my patients with hypoglycemia, protein at breakfast in addition to high-fiber foods such as steel-cut oats prevents hypoglycemia in the afternoon after lunch. It is equally important to eat a well-balanced breakfast as well as a healthy lunch to prevent cortisol dysregulation.

Many cultures, not influenced by the food industry, eat a breakfast that satisfies what the body really needs. The Japanese often have fish products and sea vegetables, while Europeans have fish such as kippers or smoked salmon. Even the much-maligned English breakfast of a boiled egg, cooked tomatoes, and toast is better than a bowl of corn flakes. Here is another radical thought I often suggest, especially if eggs are not appropriate because of allergy or elevated cholesterol: eat dinner at breakfast. Make enough dinner for two meals and have leftovers if time is short in the morning.

Other ideas for breakfast include steel-cut oatmeal (slow cooking) with walnuts, almonds, and flaxseed powder, or a serving of low fat yogurt. Add berries and other fruits and a slice of whole grain bread or brown rice cake with almond butter to round out the protein, complex carbohydrates, and essential fatty acids. Eggs, boiled, poached or over- easy, cooked without breaking the yolks (when the cholesterol in the yolk is directly exposed to high temperatures it becomes oxidized and is injurious to arterial walls), generally do not raise cholesterol. If concerned regarding cholesterol, use egg whites instead. Low-fat yogurt or goat-milk yogurt is a quick and easy protein source. Smoked salmon, herring, or tuna can all be used if the idea of kippers does not seem enticing. Well-designed protein powder, based in whey, soy, or rice is another alternative source that works especially well with children and teenagers.

What about that cup of coffee that is part of breakfast for so many people? Studies have shown that caffeine raises cortisol and epinephrine levels, especially in people at higher risk for hypertension. In one study, cortisol levels were assessed at rest and sixty minutes after continuous work on a mental stressor and a psychometric task. Findings showed an increased elevation in cortisol response when combining caffeine and the stressful task. This was true in both groups but even more exaggerated in the group at higher risk for hypertension.

In another study, caffeine was shown to increase ACTH from the pituitary leading to a greater cortisol response. However, recent data has also demonstrated a beneficial effect of coffee consumption on prevention of Type 2 diabetes. Researchers found that the amount of caffeine typically found in a cup of espresso inhibited 11 beta-hydroxysteroid dehydrogenase (11beta-HSD1) activity. This is the same enzyme found to have increased activity in obese patients, raising cortisol levels in fat cells. Whether it is the caffeine or a polyphenol in the coffee that has this effect is not clear. My suggestion is that one cup of coffee per day can be used by obese patients or those at low risk for activating the adrenal response or hypertension.

Another important eating pattern, especially if low blood sugar or the need for weight loss is an issue, is to have protein rich snacks between meals. Eating every three hours will maintain normal blood sugar, prevent the breakdown of muscle protein, and keep insulin levels under control. Nut butters, seeds and nuts, yogurts, or other easily accessible foods are good choices for midmeal snacks.

The Adaptation Diet Outline

Following is an outline for the cortisol controlling Adaptation Diet:
What to include:
- The largest portion of every meal should be vegetables, with grains and animal protein in smaller amounts.

- Use one cup of cruciferous vegetables per day (broccoli, Brussels sprouts, kale, cauliflower, and cabbage), and liberally use onions, shallots, and garlic.
- Have at least one vegetarian dinner every week.
- Use one cup of beans (kidney, navy, mung, lima, lentils, split peas) five times a week—they are a great source of fiber, complex carbohydrates, and omega 3 fats.
- Eat organically grown foods whenever possible, including free-range chicken and eggs
- Avoid hypoglycemia by eating a protein-rich breakfast and using only protein-rich snacks (nuts and nut butters, low-fat yogurt, soy products) between meals.
- Drink juice with organic green vegetables including kale, Swiss chard, and spinach mixed with carrots at least three days a week. It's best to use a machine that keeps the pulp with the juice rather than extracting the juice.
- Include anti-inflammatory and membrane-stabilizing fats—omega 3 fatty acids from walnuts, flaxseeds, pepitas, beans, salmon, herring, tuna, and sardines, and monounsaturated fats from olive oil, almonds, avocado, hazelnuts, and canola oil (cook only with olive, grapeseed, or canola oil).
- Have at least three portions of fish a week (wild salmon, anchovies, herring, mackerel, sardines, sturgeon, low-mercury tuna).
- Use two tablespoons a day of fresh ground organic flaxseed powder on salads or cereals (flax lignans reduce cortisol overproduction and detoxify hormones).
- Supplement with at least 1000 mg of EPA-DHA fish oil capsules on days that no fish is eaten to control excess cortisol production.
- Incorporate colorful vegetables (carrots, squash, cabbage, tomatoes, etc.) and fruits (blueberries, pomegranate, and cherries for example) rich in flavonoids and carotenoids in every meal with at least seven portions per day.
- Eggs should come from free-range and organically fed chickens and cooked without breaking the yolk (boiled, poached, fried over easy), or as an alternative use egg whites only.
- Use herbs and spices that are anti-inflammatory and detoxifying—turmeric, cardamom, cilantro, ginger, onion, garlic, parsley.
- Liberally use flavonoid-rich detoxifying vegetables including shiitake and ganoderma mushrooms, broccoli, tomatoes, arugula, chard, kale, spinach, and other dark greens. Cooked tomato products protect against prostate disease in men.

- Foods rich in flavonoids include green tea, cherries, blueberries, red grapes, beets, legumes, asparagus, purple onions, sweet potatoes, and spices such as ginger, parsley, sage, and turmeric. Other potent members of the flavonoid group include rutin in buckwheat, hesperidin in citrus fruits, silymarin in milk thistle, genistein in soybeans, and apigenin in chamomile.
- Drink one half (in ounces) of your body weight in filtered water every day. For example, if you weigh 130 pounds, drink 65 ounces of water. This will reduce aldosterone levels, help with weight loss, and normalize blood pressure.
- Choose green tea over black tea or coffee as a hot beverage. Black tea contains fewer catechins and the polyphenol EGCG.
- Use soy products rich in genestein and diadzein in the form of miso, tofu, edamame, and tempeh to detoxify hormones and protect cell membranes.
- Maintain a healthy weight to reduce inflammation and leptin resistance (even the loss of 5–10 percent of body weight changes cortisol and leptin levels).
- Supplement with probiotics (beneficial bacteria including lactobacillus and bifidobacter) especially after antibiotic use.
- Snack with protein-rich foods and never with high-glycemic carbohydrates as they will trigger more hypoglycemia. Nut butters, nuts, seeds, and low-fat yogurts are a few ideas for good snacks. Adding protein between meals can help with weight management and maintenance of good muscle mass.
- Strive for 25 grams of fiber per day from beans, whole grains, vegetables, flaxseed powder, or supplemental products such as psyllium seeds to reduce harmful bacteria in the gut and promote healthy bacteria that reduces inflammation and removes toxins from the body.

What to avoid:

- Avoid foods identified as allergy triggers (as documented in Phase Two) for three months. (If unclear about which foods to eliminate, avoid for one month the following trigger foods: wheat, sugar, eggs, dairy products, corn, beef, tomatoes, soy, chocolate, coffee, alcohol. These can be reintroduced one per day after avoidance, observing for reactions.)
- Avoid hypoglycemia by eating a protein-rich breakfast and using only protein-rich snacks between meals.

- Limit pro-inflammatory saturated fats (red meat, pork, lamb, poultry skin, whole dairy products, tropical oils) and omega 6 vegetable oils (corn, soy, sunflower, safflower, cottonseed, and peanut).
- Eliminate all trans fats (hydrogenated and partially hydrogenated vegetable oils).
- Eliminate gluten grains, especially in breads and baked goods (wheat, barley, and rye), for three months and use in limited amount after that (most people can use steel cut oats as a cereal, which is a good source of fiber, and brown rice as their primary grain).
- Limit high-glycemic-index foods (see appendix section 1), and emphasize fiber rich carbohydrates such as beans and root vegetables.
- Reduce caffeine intake to one cup of coffee or black tea per day to reduce inflammation and cortisol levels and prevent elevated cholesterol and homocysteine. Avoid all colas. Use green tea as the primary hot beverage.
- Moderate alcohol consumption—no more than one drink every other day for women and one drink per day for men, preferably red wine or beer that contains polyphenols such as resveratrol, which reduces inflammation.

Maintaining control over inflammation is a major step toward healthy aging. Diet is the single most important factor in reducing inflammation and normalizing cortisol levels. Pro-inflammatory foods need to be avoided and anti-inflammatory foods included.

Table 1: Pro-inflammatory Villains to Avoid

- Cold cuts, bacon, hot dogs, canned meats, sausages
- Pork, beef (organically fed and free range is better), eggs (except organic and free range no more than four per week, preferably egg whites)
- All trans fats in baked goods, chips, cake mixes, crackers, fried foods, shortenings, hydrogenated and partially hydrogenated vegetable oils
- All deep fried foods
- Whole dairy except organically fed cows (low or moderate amounts of cultured dairy such as yogurt and kefir are acceptable)
- Polyunsaturated oils (peanut, safflower, sunflower, soy, corn) and lard
- White flour, white sugar products including cookies, baked goods, candy, ice creams, ketchup, and other condiments
- Caffeinated coffee, colas, soft drinks, sweetened fruit drinks, black teas

Table 2: Anti-inflammatory Good Guys

- Vegetables—asparagus, beets, broccoli, Brussels sprouts, cabbage, carrots, cauliflower, celery, chard, bean sprouts, kale, spinach, lettuces (not iceberg), red onions, garlic, avocadoes (actually a fruit), cooked tomatoes, red and yellow peppers, squash, zucchini, sweet potatoes, yams
- Legumes—soybeans (best as edamame, tempeh, tofu, miso soup), green beans, navy beans, mung beans, lentils, split peas, white beans, black beans (never refried beans)
- Fruits—red grapes, blackberries, cranberries, red currants, blueberries, cherries, apples, pears, plums, pineapple, mangoes, tangerines, grapefruit, oranges
- Herbs—turmeric, parsley, sage, rosemary, thyme, basil, mint, ginger
- Protein—wild salmon, anchovies, herring, sardines, tuna (low mercury), mackerel, tilapia, cod, red snapper, organically raised poultry
- Nuts and seeds (best raw and unsalted, can be used as nut butters)—almonds, flaxseeds (best if ground), shelled pumpkin seeds, walnuts, pepitas, sunflower seeds, sesame seeds (tahini)
- Grains—buckwheat, brown rice, millet, quinoa, steel cut oats, smaller amounts of corn, whole wheat, rye
- Beverages—green tea, red wine (limit to one glass per day), herbal teas

In addition to the effects of phytonutrients in foods—such as flavonoids and other polyphenols, and carotenoids on inflammation and controlling cortisol—vitamin C, vitamin E, zinc, copper, selenium, and other minerals and vitamins also play a major role in normalizing cortisol and enhancing adaptation.

The appendix (section 3) contains recipes to put the Adaptation Diet into action.

Choosing Organically Raised Foods

For decades I have been a strong proponent of eating organically grown foods. After spending many years studying and becoming board certified in environmental medicine, I found alarming evidence of the sheer volume of man-made chemicals allowed in the food chain. Pesticides, herbicides, and fungicides are a major source of premature aging. All of these chemicals have a toxic effect and require the body's concerted effort to detoxify itself. This leads to greater oxidant stress and increases the need for cortisol to reduce the subsequent inflammation, triggering the aging effect of elevated cortisol levels.

However, I have recently discovered another major link between pesticide use, cancer risk, and premature aging. Several researchers have found that the health-protecting properties of foods like broccoli and berries are severely diminished through the plants' contact with pesticides. In broccoli for example, the active phytonutrient (glucosinolate or sulfurophane), a proven anticancer agent, exists as a natural pesticide to protect the broccoli plant from insects. However, this life-giving nutrient is deactivated when the plant is exposed to man-made pesticides. Unfortunately, the same effect of pesticides is found in other foods rich in anti-aging nutrients including berries, grapes, chard, kale, and spinach. This process is repeated throughout the vegetable kingdom reducing the anti-aging benefits associated with use of flavonoid and carotenoid-rich vegetables and fruits. The exception is organically raised produce.

Luckily, organic produce is now widely available. Taking it one step further, freshly harvested produce has the highest content of polyphenols and flavonoids. To ensure the most nutritious vegetables and fruits, I suggest to my patients that they buy their organically grown produce at a local farmer's market when possible. Otherwise, health-oriented supermarkets have a wide variety of organic produce.

I also suggest the use of organically produced dairy products, fowl, meat, and eggs when possible. As I mentioned earlier, the essential fatty acid content of eggs is dramatically better in free-range and organically fed chickens. If red meat is to be used, look for grass-fed free-range cattle, which have lower levels of harmful fatty acids like the arachidonic acid found in the beef. Especially with beef, but also with chicken, organically raised animals will not have the extra burden of antibiotics, growth hormones, pesticide residues, and other harmful chemicals that have made their way to the dinner table via the typical industrial farming techniques.

Chapter Six
The Stars of the Adaptation Diet

The maintenance of allostasis and adaptation depends on making good choices at the dinner table. Understanding the science of adaptation makes it easier to stay with the Adaptation Diet and create eating habits that fit each person's lifestyle. This chapter contains details about the beneficial effects of foods rich in phytonutrients that decrease inflammation, prevent free radical damage, protect cell membranes, and decrease the impact of toxins. All of these foods and phytonutrients protect the midbrain and brain from damage and reduce allostatic load and the need for cortisol production. These foods form the basis of the Adaptation Diet. The major groups of these adaptive superstars are carotenoids, flavonoids, polyphenols, and isoflavones.

Carotenoids

I remember bringing my children to an exhibit at Epcot Center in Disneyworld and seeing a kitchen come to life with dancing and singing by the different food groups as well as the appliances. (Sadly this is no longer one of the shows at Epcot.) The line that caught my attention was "Remember, vegetables are your friends." It certainly is true that the vegetable world is packed full of life protecting and detoxifying nutrients, including the carotenoids. These critical antioxidants are found in yellow, orange, red, and green vegetables as well as tomatoes, sweet potatoes, sea vegetables such as kelp, and squash.

There are over six hundred carotenoids in the food chain with new compounds being isolated seemingly every month. They all protect cell membranes against free radical damage from toxins, protecting the heart, prostate, breast, liver, and other vital organs. For example, lycopene, a potent antioxidant that gives tomatoes their red color, is effective in scavenging free radicals in cell membranes and preventing oxidation of lipoproteins (the proteins that carry fat such as cholesterol through the blood) and reducing the incidence of prostate and breast cancer and heart disease. Lutein and zeaxanthin, carotenoids found in dark green vegetables such as spinach and kale, are the chief constituents of the macular pigment in the eye and protect against adult macular degeneration, the leading cause of blindness in older Americans. These carotenoids might also protect against heart disease and other vascular problems.

Beta-carotene, the most thoroughly studied carotenoid, a precursor for vitamin A and an important antioxidant in its own right, is found in greatest amounts in yellow and orange vegetables such as carrots, squash, sweet potatoes, and yams. Beta-carotene appears to accumulate in arterial plaque and might protect against heart disease. It has been shown to retard cancer in certain animal studies.

However in human studies, supplementation of beta-carotene alone (with no other antioxidants given) in cigarette smokers demonstrated a slight increase in the incidence of smoking-related cancers. The most likely reason was the lack of other antioxidants provided to these patients. Beta-carotene, vitamin E, vitamin C, and other nutrients work as a team to detoxify free radicals and protect DNA and cellular membranes. Excessive use of any antioxidant causes a relative deficiency in the others. In addition, beta-carotene needs to be combined with the other carotenoids to be protective.

The average daily intake of carotenoids for adult women in the United States has been estimated to total 6 mg per day. However, optimum intake of beta-carotene itself is estimated to be 9–12 mg, while the typical average intake is only 1.8 mg. The average intake of the other carotenoids is estimated in the following table. These are all inadequate amounts to ensure detoxification and cell protection. The following table is a guide to foods rich in carotenoids and details how much is currently used on average in a typical American diet. The Adaptation Diet calls for much greater intake of all these foods.

Table 1: Carotenoid Intake in a Typical American Diet

Total carotenoids	6.0 mg/day	
Category	*Intake (mg)*	*Dietary Sources*
Beta carotene	1.8	Carrots, cantaloupe, broccoli, tomatoes, apricots, green peppers, leafy greens, spinach, squash, and sweet potatoes

Alpha carotene	0.4	Carrots, tomatoes, apples, corn, green peppers, leafy greens, peaches, potatoes, squash, and watermelon
Lycopene	2.6	Tomato products, watermelon, apricots, carrots, green peppers, and pink grapefruit
Lutein/zeaxanthin	1.3	Spinach, green leafy vegetables, and broccoli
B-cryptoxanthin	0.03	Oranges, tangerines, apples, apricots, corn, green peppers, lemons, papayas, and persimmons

Flavonoids

Another major group of important antioxidants is the flavonoids. There are over four thousand flavonoids in the diet, mostly found in fruits and vegetables, herbs and spices. The flavonoids provide the dark color to the skin of vegetables and fruits, such as the color of red onions. Americans consume about one fifth the amount of flavonoids as Asians, explaining in part the lower incidence of cancer and heart disease in people with traditional Asian diets compared to Americans. Total flavonoid intake is inversely related to the incidence of heart disease.

The flavonoids include catechins from green tea; polyphenols from red grape skin found in wine, which protect against heart disease; and quercitin, a potent antioxidant in grapefruits that helps regenerate vitamin C. Foods richest in flavonoids include legumes, green tea, cherries, blueberries, raspberries, red grapes, beets, asparagus, onions, sweet potatoes, and spices such as ginger, parsley, sage, and turmeric as well as many Chinese and Ayeurvedic herbal remedies. Other potent members of the flavonoid group include rutin in buckwheat, hesperidin in citrus fruits, silymarin in milk thistle, genistein in soybeans, apigenin in chamomile, and resveratrol in red grapes and wine.

A superstar of the flavonoids is green tea, produced by lightly steaming the leaves of the tea plant (*Camellia sinensis*). Polyphenols, the biologically active compounds in teas, are partially deactivated when tea is oxidized (black tea). The polyphenols in green tea include catechin, proanthocyanadins, and epigallocatechin, considered the most active flavonoid in tea.

In experimental studies, the green tea polyphenols have shown higher antioxidant activity than vitamin C and vitamin E. Green tea can also increase the activity of detoxifying enzymes including glutathione and catalase, active in the liver, lungs, and small intestine. Green tea activates both Phase One and Phase Two detoxification.

Studies have shown that green tea consumption reduces the incidence of many cancers including stomach, small intestine, bladder, prostate, skin, pancreas, colon, breast, and lung. The lower incidence of cancer in Japan might be explained at least in part by green tea consumption. Green tea appears to inhibit estrogen's stimulation of breast receptors in estrogen-sensitive cancers. Additionally, green tea suppresses the activation of carcinogens, detoxifies carcinogens, and inhibits nitrosamine production from foods such as bacon, hot dogs, ham, and other processed meat.

In most of these studies, green tea consumption was four to ten cups per day. Each cup contains an average of 80–120 mg of polyphenols. Green tea extracts can be used that contain 300 to 400 mg of polyphenols standardized to contain 80 percent polyphenols and 55 percent epigallocatechin. To reach the possible benefit found in population studies, a minimum of 300 mg should be taken as a supplement.

Studies have shown remarkable properties in another underutilized food: wild blueberries. In animal studies, rats fed wild blueberries had better memory for spatial tasks and improved coordination. During World War II, British pilots ate wild blueberries to improve their night vision and coordination. Blueberries contain high amounts of polyphenols that give the berries their blue color and tartness. These chemicals have been shown to be strong antioxidants that are cardioprotective, improve circulation, inhibit certain cancers, and protect against age-related cognitive dysfunction and motor deficits. It appears that the more tart wild blueberry has a higher concentration of these polyphenols than those commercially produced. In either case, these studies show the benefit of eating a wide variety of fruits and vegetables, especially those with intense coloration including pomegranate, raspberries, blackberries, and red grapes.

Quercitin, one of the most potent flavonoids, has been shown to protect against the development of diabetic complications such as diabetic cataracts, neuropathy, and retinopathy. Quercitin also appears to have potent antiviral properties, as do most of the flavonoids. Studies have shown inhibition of viral infections including herpes type 1, para influenza, polio, and respiratory syncytial virus. Quercitin might also have some benefit in treating the common cold. The recommended dosage as a supplement is 200–400 mg taken twenty minutes before a meal. It is also helpful to take bromelain, a digestive enzyme from pineapple with the quercitin, to enhance its anti-inflammatory effect.

Proanthocyanadins, which are found in grape seeds, red wine, and commercial extracts from maritime pine bark, have potent antioxidant and anti-inflammatory effects. They prevent damage to collagen, the protein that comprises much of the connective tissue, tendons, and ligaments. These potent antioxidants have fifty times the effect in protecting connective tissue than does vitamin C and can reduce symptoms from arthritis and allergies, lower cholesterol, strengthen capillaries, and promote healthy skin.

Soybeans and Isoflavones

Soy protects against heart disease and stroke, lowers cholesterol, and protects against hormonally influenced cancers such as breast and prostate. Soy products, including tofu, soybeans (edamame), miso, soy milk, tempeh, and soy nuts contain the isoflavones genestein, equol, diadzein, and others that are critical in the detoxification process and reduce the effect of hormones on receptors. They lower inflammation by reducing levels of inflammatory mediators, C-reactive protein, TNF alpha, and interleukin-6. They also enhance detoxification of estrogen and testosterone, one reason for the very low incidence in Asia of breast cancer and menopausal symptoms. Genestein and the other soy isoflavones influence the synthesis of tumor proteins, slow the growth of malignant cells, block procancer enzymes, and inhibit the growth of blood vessels that nourish tumors.

In women who are low in estrogen, such as in menopause, soy isoflavone stimulation of estrogen receptors can reduce symptoms of menopause significantly. Many of my patients can reduce hot flashes by using miso, tempeh, and tofu products. The fermented soy products are higher in genestein and might provide greater detoxification and protection against hormonally induced disease. If needed, I recommend consuming one serving of soy per day. That's about three ounces of tofu or ½ cup of tempeh or miso. I don't recommend soy milk as a source of these isoflavones because it is not a food that was part of traditional Oriental diets and has never been studied long term. There has been much controversy over the negative effects of excess soy products on breast health and thyroid function. Using only fermented traditional sources of soy reduces these risks and is an appropriate food choice.

Other foods that contain smaller amounts of these isoflavones are the other legumes, alfalfa, clover, licorice root, and kudzu root. Kudzu root has been used in supplements in place of soy in soy allergic patients.

Legumes

If there is one group of foods that most Americans underutilize, it is legumes. These nutritional powerhouses are a perfect blend of soluble and insoluble fiber, essential fatty acids, protein, and complex carbohydrates. They contain phytohormones, lignans, and isoflavonoids, which provide cancer protection and lower LDL cholesterol and act to detoxify hormones and toxins. Because of their fiber properties, they stabilize blood sugar levels, preventing obesity and type 2 diabetes. The legumes include soybeans, kidney beans, lentils, adzuki beans, black beans, brown beans, chickpeas, mung beans, navy beans, pinto beans, red beans, and split peas. One cup of cooked beans per day is a worthy goal.

Cruciferous Vegetables

Your mother was right when she told you to eat your broccoli. Broccoli is one of the cruciferous (Brassica family) vegetables, an essential food group for detoxification and healthy aging. Other crucifers include cauliflower, Brussels sprouts, cabbage, bok choy, kale, mustard greens, rutabaga, turnips, and watercress. They induce several enzyme systems including glutathione S transferase and glutathione peroxidase that are potent cell membrane protectors. The compounds in these foods include aryl isothiocyanates and indole 3 carbinol, which detoxifies estrogen, protecting against breast and prostate cancer. Animals fed cruciferous vegetables and then exposed to the deadly carcinogen aflatoxin had a 90 percent reduction in the incidence of cancer. Smokers that chewed two ounces of watercress at each meal had a significant increase in the detoxification of nicotine compared to controls. Because indoles are easily destroyed during cooking, either steam your crucifers or eat them raw.

Cruciferous vegetables are rich in glucosinolates that enhance glutathione levels and increase detoxification. Glutathione is a key antioxidant that protects cell membranes from oxidative damage. An overload of toxins from poor diet, alcohol, cigarettes, or over the counter medication can deplete glutathione and pose risks for cancer and inflammatory processes.

Turmeric

A good example of the potency of spices and herbs is turmeric, used in Indian cooking for centuries. It contains curcumin, a potent antioxidant that influences cell signaling pathways. Turmeric inhibits the inflammatory process and reduces the need for cortisol production, lowers total cholesterol, raises

HDL, and prevents abnormal clotting. Turmeric reduces lipid peroxides, a measure of oxidant stress, and protects lipids from oxidation. This spice is found in prepared mustard and as a supplement.

Methionine and Cysteine

Amino acids, the building blocks of protein, are used in the detoxification process. The most important of these are the sulfur containing amino acids, cysteine and methionine, which lead to glutathione manufacture, a compound that detoxifies and acts as a powerful antioxidant. Glutathione levels can be increased through the use of meats, nuts, asparagus, and avocados. However, glutathione is easily destroyed by the use of alcohol, acetaminophen, and other drugs. Vitamin C at 500 mg can protect glutathione from degradation. N-acetylcyteine, available as a supplement, increases glutathione levels and can treat toxicity from drugs such as acetaminophen as well as from environmental toxins.

Foods that are rich in the sulfur amino acids methionine and cysteine include eggs, fish, dairy products, poultry, beans, nuts, and seeds. The more environmental stress from toxins and drugs, the higher the need for these foods to provide the sulfur as a building block for detoxification. The sulfur amino acids also are the key factors in sulfation, which converts many toxic intermediates into harmless substances.

Garlic

Garlic has been used for five thousand years as a medicinal food. It was noted by Pasteur that garlic was an antiseptic. It has long been used as an antiparasitic in many cultures throughout the world. Recent evidence shows that garlic has immune-system-stimulating properties as well. White blood cells from people fed garlic were able to kill 139 percent more tumor cells than non-garlic users. In another study, mice were protected from the development of tumors through feeding with garlic. In a study of 1600 people in China, high intake of garlic reduced stomach cancer rates by 50 percent.

A clove of garlic is a gold mine of phytonutrients with more than thirty different active compounds that detoxify and protect against free radical damage. (Chives, leeks, onions, and shallots also contain many of these nutrients.) These include the sulfur-containing phytonutrients allylic sulfides (thiols), allicin and ajoene, saponins and phenolics. These substances have been shown to lower cholesterol; reduce the stickiness of blood platelets; act as natural antibiotics against viruses, bacteria, fungi, and parasites; and block tumor growth. In a study in AIDS patients, those taking 5–10 grams of aged garlic (equivalent to three small cloves) developed a higher functioning immune system as measured by natural killer cell activity.

Garlic (as well as onions) also contains flavonoid compounds including quercitin, which have anti-carcinogenic effects. These are potent antioxidants associated with reduced risk of skin cancer, leukemia, and experimentally induced cancers in rodents.

Table 2: Phytochemicals that Improve Detoxification

Compound	Source
isothiocyanates	cruciferous vegetables(broccoli, cabbage, kale)
glucosinolates	cruciferous vegetables
organosulfurs	garlic, onions
curcumin	turmeric
flavonoids	numerous fruits and vegetables
monoterpenes	citrus peel

Mushrooms

The medicinal use of mushrooms such as maitake, reishi (*ganaderma lucidum*), enoki, and shiitake (*lentinus edodes*) is highly developed in the Orient. These mushrooms have strong effects on enhancing immune function including natural killer cell activity and inhibiting tumor growth. Oral extract of maitake, which contains beta-glucan, a polysaccharide, has been shown by Shomori (*Oncology Reports,* 2009) to have potential antitumor effects in gastric cancer cell lines.

The dose needed to stimulate the immune response is 900 mg per day. Shiitake is available in many food stores and can readily be added to meals. I also have my patients use an alcohol tincture of a mixture of ganaderma, shiitake, and cordyceps sinensis for acute viral illness. For people who need immune enhancement for chronic illness, these mushrooms can be used in capsule form. A typical combination includes *cordyceps, ganoderma, coriolus versicolor, lentinus edode* (shiitake*) and grifola frondosus.*

Yogurt, Beneficial Bacteria and Colostrum

Yogurt is often overlooked as an adaptogenic food because of the number of people who avoid dairy products. Other than those people with a dairy allergy or severe lactose intolerance, yogurt and kefir can be extremely beneficial. In traditional cultures such as the Hunzas in the Caucasus Mountains of Central

Europe, cultured dairy products, which form the basis of their diets, have been linked to longevity and a reduced incidence of heart disease.

Yogurt and kefir are fermented dairy products that contain active cultures of lactobacillus and bifidobacter bacteria (probiotics). These and other types of healthy gut bacteria number in the trillions but are affected by antibiotic use, alcohol, poor diet, stress, and toxins in the diet. Reduced levels of healthy gut bacteria have been implicated in chronic inflammation of the digestive tract and lower immunity against infection.

Probiotics play a major role in regulating allergic reactions to foods and reducing inflammation through suppressing growth of abnormal bacteria and yeasts. These beneficial bacteria aid in the detoxification of hormones and other chemicals and prevent reabsorption of antigens and chemicals that trigger inflammation. They inhibit the formation of carcinogens from dietary sources and enhance immune function. In addition, they produce vitamins B and K and are necessary for healthy clotting and nervous system function.

In studies using yogurt with live cultures (check the label to make sure there are live cultures), many immune system effects have been shown including tripling of interferon production, raising the activity of the natural killer cells (the cells that destroy potential cancer cells), and blocking the effect of carcinogenic agents in the colon on the development of colon cancer. In a study of 1000 women with breast cancer, there was an inverse relationship between the amount of yogurt consumed and the incidence of breast cancer. Yogurt is best used without added sweeteners, especially aspartame. Blended yogurts with high amounts of fructose should also be avoided.

Two of the active ingredients found in breast milk, colostrum and lactoferrin, are also potent immune enhancers and regulators. These protein molecules are peptides that directly affect the function of the immune system and defend against invasive organisms. Lactoferrin bonds to iron in the digestive tract and destroys bacteria that are dependent on iron as a nutrient. Colostrum is a peptide that regulates the immune response. In cases of immune deficiency such as cancer or AIDS, colostrum can enhance the function of the immune response. When used by individuals with autoimmune disease such as rheumatoid arthritis, colostrum appears to reduce the immune system's attack on native tissues.

To increase healthy adaptation, I often suggest supplementation with probiotics and colostrum products. There are several strains of lactobacillus especially effective against abnormal gut organisms: lactobacillus GG, lactobacillus rhaminosis, and lactobacillus acidophilus NCFM. Strains of bifidobacter also regulate the health of the small intestine and should be included in any supplement program. It is important that the manufacturer guarantees the potency of the strain to contain at least ten billion organisms per capsule. Most need to be refrigerated to maintain potency. Colostrum and lactoferrin are also available as supplements.

Protecting the Amygdala and Hippocampus through Nutritional Supplements and the Adaptogenic Diet

When all is said and done, one of the most important goals of proper dietary habits is to protect the brain from damage induced by elevated cortisol and oxidant stress. Food-based nutrients are the cornerstone of preserving normal cell membrane health. However, with the stress patterns that I see in my patients as well as the pollutants from the environment and the food chain, using nutritional supplementation targeted at protecting the neurons of the midbrain is often required.

Cortisol and epinephrine increase lipid peroxidation and cause damage to cell membranes from free radicals including singlet oxygen, super oxide, and hydrogen peroxide. Injury can be to the cell membrane, the DNA, or the mitochondria, the energy-producing-organelles inside the cell. Protecting against this damage are antioxidant molecules that are either made in the body or derived from food and supplements.

Stress, poor adaptation, and elevated cortisol age the brain. Aging itself increases cortisol and its damaging effect on the cerebral cortex and the hippocampus, which is intimately involved with memory and mood. Damage to the hippocampus alters the feedback control of cortisol production making the situation even worse. This leads to early memory loss, depression, anxiety, and fatigue.

Table 3: Effects of Elevated Cortisol on Brain Aging

- Increases inflammatory hormone gene expression (5-lipoxygenase)
- Increases nerve sensitivity to toxins and poor blood flow
- Inhibits testosterone, estrogen and growth hormone secretion
- Affects mood and behavior
- Permanently down regulates hippocampal cell receptors
- Alters neurotransmitter function
- Disrupts memory recall and cognition
- Increases insulin resistance
- Promotes neuronal cell atrophy, injury, and death
- Promotes failure of the mitochondrial mechanism and neurotoxicity

Protecting the brain from damage should be everyone's number-one priority. The Adaptation Diet, stress reduction through meditation and relaxation techniques, exercise, and changes in attitude and behavior are all needed to improve adaptation. In addition, several nutrients have been shown to be neuroprotective through specific membrane-sparing effects, preventing free-radical damage to the brain from allostatic load. These include alpha lipoic acid, which improves healthy glucose transport and metabolism and promotes function of the mitochondria, the cellular energy factory. Lipoic acid is a potent antioxidant and helps regenerate vitamin C and vitamin E, particularly in the nervous-system tissue.

Alpha lipoic acid improves energy production through ATP synthesis. It is a strong antioxidant and acts as a chelator of heavy metals. It increases the synthesis of glutathione, the most important antioxidant found in brain tissue, and scavenges reactive oxygen species (its antioxidant effect). It works both inside and outside the cells of the nervous system. It improves the removal of glucose from the bloodstream, increasing insulin receptor sensitivity. In patients with diabetic neuropathy, 800–1200 mg per day has been used with positive results. For nondiabetic individuals, a time-released preparation in the amount of 400–800 mg per day is suggested.

Other key brain nutrients include acetyl-l-carnitine; N-acetyl-cysteine; carotenoids including lutein and resveratrol (from grapes); the B vitamins especially B6, B12, and folic acid (critical for methylation to detoxify toxins); coenzyme Q10 for mitochondrial function and antioxidant effect; ginkgo biloba for improved blood flow and antioxidant protection; EPA-DHA (cold-water fish oils especially from salmon and tuna) for support of the membranes of the brain cells; and vitamin E including both alpha and gamma tocopherol.

Acetyl-l-carnitine is a nonessential amino acid derivative and improves mitochondrial energy production. In several studies it has been shown to improve cognitive function and delay the onset of dementia. It also increases the production of acetycholine, a critical neurotransmitter. Carnitine can also clear abnormal deposition of fatty acids and has been shown to decrease triglyceride levels. Acetyl-l-carnitine is more active in the brain than carnitine itself. Doses used in the studies in dementia ranged from 1.5 to 3 grams.

Magnesium is needed for normal mitochondrial function in the production of energy. It is depleted when glucose is elevated from increased cortisol levels. Elevated intakes of dietary fats and calcium also deplete magnesium stores. Magnesium is needed for normal muscle tone and is useful in the treatment of asthma, migraine, anxiety, and muscle spasm. In patients with chronic pain, magnesium levels are often depleted and cause additional lack of stress resistance. The best form of magnesium is citrate with a dose of 300–500 mg per day.

Coenzyme Q10 is protective of brain and heart cells through its antioxidant effect and improved mitochondrial function. CoQ10 has a sparing effect on vitamin E while vitamin E allows CoQ10 to be more effective when taken as a supplement. A dose of 150 mg was shown to improve brain function in Parkinson's patients. CoQ10 also showed significant effects in improving cardiac function in patients with cardiomyopathy. (One third of the heart weight is comprised of mitochondria, which are dependent upon adequate CoQ10 levels.) Doses should be at least 100 mg of a crystalline-free oil-based preparation.

Table 4: CoQ10 Facts

- Protects against cholesterol oxidation
- Found in organ meats
- Decreases after age forty leading to decreased mitochondrial function
- Useful in atrial fibrillation, CHF, MVP, hypertension
- Decreases angina and ST depression
- Improves exercise tolerance, reduces LDL oxidation
- All patients on statin drugs should supplement with at least 100 mg per day of CoQ10.

N-Acetylcysteine (NAC) has a potent antioxidant effect through increasing levels of glutathione (GSH), the key cellular antioxidant. Glutathione also increases disposal of peroxides and protects cell membranes and the nucleus. NAC has been shown to increase electron transport in the mitochondria and activates enzymes to increase energy production from the mitochondria. There is also evidence of reduction of cell death or apoptosis with the use of NAC. Doses of NAC should range from 100–500 mg per day.

Vitamin E is the primary fat-soluble antioxidant found in all tissues. Low levels lead to higher risk for degenerative diseases of the brain such as Alzheimer's and Parkinson's. It is protective against the oxidative stress effects of elevated cortisol levels. High doses of vitamin E up to 2000 IU per day have been shown to slow the onset of progression of Alzheimer's by up to two years. Mixed tocopherols including both the gamma and alpha forms are more consistent with what is found in food and should be the only form of vitamin E used as supplement. Blood levels of vitamin E are also predictive of heart disease with the lowest levels showing an increased risk of developing coronary artery disease. In fact, vitamin E levels are a more important predictor of heart disease than are cholesterol levels. For brain protection, 200–800 mg of mixed tocopherols are suggested. (Recent studies have shown that using high doses of one antioxidant such as vitamin E without corresponding doses of other antioxidants such as vitamin C can be harmful. I always recommend a mixed antioxidant supplement that contains adequate amounts of mixed tocopherols, vitamin C, and carotenoids.)

Table 5: Food Sources of Vitamin E

- Almonds
- Asparagus
- Avocado
- Olive oil
- Wheat germ
- Soybeans

Niacinamide (vitamin B3) helps maintain normal blood sugar levels in people prone to hypoglycemic reactions. Niacinamide is a potent inhibitor of inflammation in the brain caused by enzymes such as nitric oxide synthetase and poly ADP-ribose polymerase (PARP). It has antioxidant effects as well as protecting mitochondrial function in the brain. Dosages of niacinamide are 100–500 mg per day.

Folate, vitamin B6, and vitamin B12 are important in detoxifying homocysteine, a product of protein metabolism that can cause vascular disease of the brain and heart. These three vitamins are needed for methylation reactions that detoxify homocysteine and protect the brain and blood vessels. Cognitive dysfunction is seen in deficiencies of these vitamins with symptoms of memory loss, forgetfulness, confusion, depression, mood changes, and dementia. Changes in stress levels and elevated cortisol can increase the requirement for these vitamins. Intake should be at least 1 mg folic acid, 25 mg B6, and 800 mcg of B12, preferably as methyl B12.

Essential fatty acids are incorporated into the tissue membranes of nerves. There is less inflammatory activity in these membranes if EPA (eicosopentaenoic acid) and DHA (docosahexaenoic acid) are substituted for arachidonic acid (from red meat, dairy, and eggs) in the membranes of the brain. These fatty acids are found in high amounts in cold-water fish such as salmon, cod, and mackerel as well as in walnuts and other nuts. The dose per day should be a minimum of 400 mg for prevention and up to 6 grams for treatment of chronic inflammation. Capsules of EPA-DHA are readily available. It is important to make sure the fish were caught in nonpolluted waters because of possible contamination with toxins from the ocean.

Resveratrol is a polyphenol found in the skins of red grapes and other plants. It is the only nutrient shown to enhance mitochondrial regeneration. In animals fed high doses of resveratrol, aging was slowed and longevity increased. Resveratrol also reduces inflammation through inhibition of COX-1, COX-2, and 5-LOX pathways. (This is the same effect of many of the common anti-inflammatory medications such as ibuprofen, aspirin, and prescription anti-inflammatory medications.) It also is a strong antioxidant and protects lipid membranes, inhibits platelet aggregation, and improves liver detoxification. Resveratrol activates the Sirtuin gene which protects the cell against damage and slows cell death. The only other activator of this gene is reduced caloric intake. Resveratrol could explain the so-called French paradox—that despite high-fat diets and large amounts of red wine, there is little heart disease in France.

Table 6: Suggested Daily Dosages for Brain Protection

- Alpha lipoic acid 400–800 mg
- Acetyl-l-carnitine 500 mg
- Coenzyme Q10 100 mg
- N-acetyl cysteine 500–1000 mg
- Vitamin E 400–800 IU of mixed tocopherols
- Vitamin C 500–1000 mg ascorbates with flavonoids
- Niacinamide 100–500 mg
- Folic acid 1 mg
- Vitamin B6 25–100 mg
- Vitamin B12 500–1000 mcg of methyl B12
- EPA-DHA 320–2000 mg of EPA

This is not meant to be an exhaustive list of supplements that might impact brain health. I suggest a good multivitamin and mineral complex in addition to some of the above nutrients. Remember that taking supplements is not a replacement for the benefits from the Adaptation Diet or good eating habits and appropriate self-care. Use of these supplements should be under the supervision of a health care professional.

Chapter Seven
Cortisol Tamers

My experience observing the wide-ranging impact of diet on my patients' ability to adapt has helped me identify several factors that directly reduce elevated cortisol levels. These include foods, herbs, vitamins, and minerals that comprise a group of substances called adaptogens. They are instrumental in managing allostasis and ensuring adaptation.

Controlling cortisol should start early in life. However, for some people childhood already presents a challenge in terms of allostatic load. Several studies have shown that maternal diet can influence the cortisol levels of children. A 2007 study looked at the children of women who had a diet containing excessive animal protein (greater than seventeen portions of meat or fish per week) and minimal amounts of carbohydrate-rich foods in the last half of pregnancy. These children had up to 46 percent higher levels of salivary cortisol in response to the Trier Test (a standardized psychological stress test). Children of women who consumed a more balanced diet using complex carbohydrates and less protein (less than thirteen portions of meat or fish per week) had significantly lower cortisol levels. In addition, there is evidence that low birth weight might also increase cortisol production and stress responsiveness later in life. Despite what may have happened in utero, there are still many things that can be done to alter cortisol levels. Following are dietary and lifestyle factors that I have found to have a significant impact on regaining adaptation.

Lose Weight and Cut Calories

Obesity itself increases cortisol levels, leading to an increased risk of metabolic syndrome, diabetes, and heart disease. The pro-aging impact of obesity is enormous in Western society, where one of every two adults is overweight and 40 percent of children are obese or overweight. A striking example of this childhood epidemic was pointed out to me on a recent ski trip. Several of the ski instructors told me that half of the young children they teach are so overweight and out of shape that they can barely get up if they fall during ski lessons! The instructors had seen a dramatic change in the number of obese children in their classes over the past five years.

Obesity stems from a combination of genetic susceptibility, diet, and lack of exercise. Diet is the number-one reason for this epidemic. Perhaps the biggest culprit is the use of refined sugars and carbohydrates and other high-glycemic-index foods, which stimulate increased appetite and craving for additional carbohydrates, greatly increasing caloric intake. Eating these foods causes an initial spike in blood sugar, followed by elevated insulin levels that then lead to lower blood sugar, increased hunger, and more food intake in an attempt to restore energy balance. Studies in both humans and animals consistently confirm these findings as underlying much of the obesity epidemic.

In a very important study of obese children, the amount of food intake was measured after the ingestion of a high-glycemic food (instant oatmeal) and compared to the intake after a low-glycemic meal (steel-cut oats). When measuring food consumption throughout the day after a breakfast and lunch of the two types of oatmeal, there was a 53 percent higher intake of calories associated with the high-glycemic food. Another study found that children allowed to eat as much low-glycemic food as they desired lost significantly more weight than those children on a diet that was low calorie and fat restricted. The bottom line is that eating high-glycemic foods markedly increases appetite and leads to a greater intake of calories throughout the day.

Certainly there are other factors contributing to the obesity epidemic including lack of exercise, high fat intake, the use of fast foods, enormous portion sizes and excess caloric intake ("supersized"), and a lack of nutrient-rich foods like legumes and cruciferous vegetables. However, the most potent pro-obesity dietary factor in the United States is the use of high-glycemic carbohydrates.

Once obesity occurs, a vicious cycle ensues of inflammation, insulin resistance, and more obesity. A person with abdominal obesity (a waist size greater than forty inches in men and thirty-five inches in women) is at much greater risk for heart disease and diabetes and metabolic syndrome. This condition includes insulin resistance as the key metabolic derangement as well as hypertension, abnormal triglycerides, and lower levels of high-density cholesterol. Twenty-five percent of obese people and 50 percent of hypertensives are insulin resistant. It is estimated that 25 percent of the U.S. population may be insulin resistant and have metabolic syndrome.

The cortisol connection appears here as well. In obese women, studies show that after eating a high carbohydrate meal, there is a marked elevation in cortisol production. This increase in cortisol often includes elevated norepinephrine levels as well and creates a maladapted response and additional allostatic load. On the other hand, a high-protein and low-carbohydrate meal does not elevate cortisol in obese women.

Obesity and excess abdominal girth themselves increase cortisol levels and interfere with adaptation. One of the most dangerous and discouraging aspects of being overweight is that once established, it is self-perpetuating. Cortisol appears to be one reason that obese people do not slim down easily. It has been shown that in the obese individual, there is a greater release of cortisol from the adrenal glands when stimulated with corticotropin-releasing hormone (CRH) from the hypothalamus and midbrain. This implies that stress from any source will cause a greater secretion of cortisol in obese people, further complicating the connection between excess weight and stress hormones and the risk for metabolic syndrome, diabetes, and heart disease.

As noted earlier, the adipocytes (fat cells, especially those in visceral fat in the abdominal cavity surrounding the internal organs) increase conversion of inactive cortisone to active cortisol through the enzyme 11HSD, resulting in elevated cortisol systemically. Amazingly, it appears that the amount of cortisol produced by this mechanism is equivalent to the amount manufactured by the adrenal system. In obesity this enzyme system in the fat cells is increased, leading to more circulating cortisol, elevated cortisol in visceral fat, and increased risk for metabolic syndrome. This makes weight loss even more challenging. In addition, the hypothalamic-pituitary-adrenal axis is activated more in obese individuals, further increasing cortisol production.

Recent findings have shown that adipocytes secrete a signaling molecule (Wnt-signaling) that directly stimulates the adrenal gland (through StAR transcription) to produce higher levels of cortisol and aldosterone, the hormone that raises blood pressure. The greater the abdominal fat, the higher the cortisol and the faster that premature aging, high blood pressure, heart disease, and diabetes occur. Obesity and increased abdominal fat also contribute to insulin resistance and a cluster of metabolic abnormalities including Type 2 diabetes, hypertension, and abnormal levels of blood fats including cholesterol and triglycerides.

If a person is overweight, there are also lower levels of the binding protein that prevents cortisol from stimulating receptor sites (corticosteroid binding globulin—CBG). This makes cortisol more available, amplifying its damaging impact. The reason the body is so intent on increasing cortisol in obesity is to attempt to reduce the chronic low level of inflammation seen in most overweight people, especially if they are eating a typical American inflammatory diet. In a study done in Spain with two hundred subjects, (Fernandez-Real, *Journal of Clinical Endocrinolgy and Metabolism,* 2002) the greater the waist-height ratio (a simple measure of obesity), the lower the CBG levels, leading to elevated free (active) cortisol. In a study from England by Steptoe (*International Journal of Obesity,* 2007), men with central obesity had morning cortisol levels that were higher than men with normal weight. Elevated morning cortisol is typically seen in high levels when stress is a major factor. It appears that simply being overweight is enough to cause maladaptation and premature aging.

Visceral abdominal fat, especially when greater than normal, functions as an endocrine organ. This startling finding flies in the face of all previous ideas about hormones and how they are produced from endocrine glands. In addition to cortisol, fat cells make leptin, a hormone that signals the brain to reduce appetite. In many cases of obesity, leptin levels become elevated because the signal is disrupted, probably from inflammatory foods, prompting more leptin production. Similar to insulin resistance, leptin resistance is associated with a chronic inflammatory state caused by dietary habits. The leptin no longer effectively shuts down appetite. Excess simple carbohydrates, the wrong fats, and too many calories all contribute to leptin resistance. The Adaptation Diet, as well as appropriate nutritional supplementation, can reduce inflammation and overcome both insulin and leptin resistance.

Visceral fat can directly increase endothelial dysfunction (a marker of the ability of blood vessels to dilate and prevent inflammatory changes leading to atherosclerosis), a major risk factor for heart disease. In a recent and important study, it was shown that as little as a nine-pound weight gain of visceral fat is associated with significant endothelial dysfunction and elevated cortisol levels. Researchers at the Mayo clinic studied forty-three lean people and put thirty-five of them on a weight gaining diet and compared them to the others who did not gain weight. They measured endothelial function through blood-flow parameters both after they gained the weight and again after they subsequently lost weight. They found impaired function of the endothelium from this modest weight gain even if blood pressure and other markers were normal, implying that even a small amount of increased visceral fat can start the process of metabolic syndrome and heart disease.

The bottom line is that even mild obesity causes inflammation leading to greater cortisol response. Studies of obese individuals show higher IL-6, NFK alpha, CRP, leptin, and insulin, all markers of inflammation. Besides releasing free fatty acids, adipocytes secrete substances that contribute to peripheral insulin resistance, including adiponectin and resistin. Increased turnover of free fatty acids interferes with intracellular metabolism of glucose in the muscle, and exerts a lipotoxic effect on pancreatic beta cells. The pre-receptor metabolism of cortisol is enhanced in visceral adipose tissue by the activation of 11 beta-hydroxysteroid dehydrogenase type 1. As noted, adipose tissue itself is the source of many of these inflammatory hormones and signaling molecules. All these changes indirectly stimulate cortisol release to reduce inflammation.

The vicious cycle of too much abdominal fat leading to elevated cortisol, which makes insulin resistance worse, leading to more weight gain, has to be broken to regain adaptation. Luckily, studies have shown that it does not take massive weight loss to regain appropriate cortisol balance. Losing as little as 5 percent of total body weight can stop the cycle of increased cortisol release and lead to adaptation. For some people 10 percent is needed, but even that is possible to accomplish with appropriate dietary changes. The majority of my patients who stay with the Adaptation Diet for at least three months, emphasizing frequent protein meals and low-glycemic carbohydrates, while eliminating allergic foods as well as glutens, sugars, and all processed foods, will lose enough weight to accomplish the goal of cortisol control. For those patients who need extra help to lose the 5 percent, supplementation with L-carnitine, alpha lipoic acid, irvingia, and green tea can jump start the process.

Of course, calorie control is also a key in weight management. Cutting calories has been proven in animal studies to be the most effective anti-aging strategy ever researched. In human studies the beneficial effect of caloric restriction has been harder to prove. In the 1990s, evidence for the efficacy of caloric restriction did appear in a most unlikely setting. Biosphere 2 was an experiment of living in a completely self-contained closed environment in the desert outside Tucson, Arizona. A self-sustaining ecological system was developed to show that humans could thrive in this setting. However, because of an unanticipated decrease in food availability, the eight men and women who lived in Biosphere 2 were forced to consume 22 percent fewer calories, while still sustaining high levels of physical activity over an eighteen-month period.

The result was a 17 percent decrease in body weight and a marked reduction in metabolic risk factors for heart disease in the Biosphere inhabitants. They had lower blood pressure, cholesterol, and glucose levels. Most interestingly, they showed lower cortisol levels and markers of inflammation such as CRP. They had higher DHEA levels, lower thyroid hormones, lower core temperature, improved insulin sensitivity, and reduced markers of oxidative stress.

Several other studies on caloric restrictions have shown additional effects on reducing inflammation, the key to aging well. Long-term human studies have not yet been done, so many scientists hesitate to tout caloric restriction as an anti-aging miracle. However, it is clear that losing weight and cutting calories, regardless of initial weight, will reduce inflammation and cortisol levels, leading to much-improved adaptation and lower allostatic loads.

Flaxseed Powder

Surprisingly, one of the most powerful regulators of cortisol production is flaxseed powder. In a study done by Spence (*Journal of the American College of Nutrition,* 2003), volunteers were fed diets containing flaxseed supplementation with differing concentrations of lignans and alpha linolenic acid. They were then given a stressful and frustrating task to perform, after which the researchers measured their levels of plasma cortisol, fibrinogen, and peripheral resistance (a marker for the elasticity of arteries). The flaxseed highest in lignans had the most significant effect in reducing plasma cortisol.

Flaxseed has been called nature's perfect food because it contains soluble fiber, omega 3 essential fatty acids, and lignans, a potent phytohormone. The omega-3 essential fatty acid is anti-inflammatory, decreasing the need for cortisol and reducing the risk for heart disease and diabetes. Lignans in flaxseeds are phytoestrogens (plant-based substances that attach to estrogen receptors, reducing stimulation from circulating hormones) and have been shown to reduce the incidence of breast and prostate cancer. In postmenopausal women with breast cancer, Canadian researchers (Thompson and Chen in *Clinical Cancer Research,* 2005) found that dietary flaxseed increased cancer cell apoptosis (cell death) and reduced tumor growth.

In a study by Prasad (*Atherosclerosis,* 2005), lignans from flaxseed reduced atherosclerosis plaques in rabbits fed a high-fat diet. The protective mechanisms of the flaxseeds included decreased oxidative stress, lower total cholesterol and LDL, and higher HDL. Lignans from flaxseeds also improved glucose control and reduced both insulin levels and insulin resistance in human volunteers.

I recommend two tablespoons of ground organic flaxseed daily, sprinkled on salads, cereals, or other foods. It is best to grind the seeds in a coffee grinder and use them right away to prevent rancidity. If you are not able to grind your own, purchase organic flaxseed powder that has vitamin E in it to prevent rancidity. Flaxseed oil capsules generally do not have the same effect unless they have added lignans.

Fish Oil and Supplements of EPA-DHA

Researchers in France (Delarue, *Diabetes Metabolism*, 2003) did one of the most important studies regarding the connection between omega-3 fatty acids and stress. They measured the stress response to mental arithmetic and other stressors before and after feeding human volunteers 7.2 grams of fish oil a day as supplements for three weeks. The measurements included plasma cortisol, catecholamine (epinephrine and norepinephrine), and non-esterified fatty acid. The response to stress, including elevations of cortisol, epinephrine, and fats was dramatically reduced by supplementation of omega-3 fatty acids. They concluded that adrenal activation could be inhibited by adequate intake of omega-3 fatty acids. The site of action is in the central nervous system. Furthermore in another paper it was postulated that essential fatty acid supplementation might reduce the injury to the hippocampus from cortisol and the subsequent development of Alzheimer's disease and other manifestation of premature aging.

Recent studies funded by the National Institutes of Health showed low dietary intake of omega-3 fats from fish promoted anger, aggression, and depression. Taking EPA-DHA supplements can reduce this effect. A study done at the Veterans Administration by Buydens-Branchey (*Psychiatry Research,* 2008) found that in male outpatients who had aggressive behavior and substance abuse showed that 3 grams of fish oil supplements (containing 2250 mg of EPA and 500 mg of DHA) reduced anger scores significantly compared to placebo. Since anger and aggression equate to high cortisol levels, this study confirms the benefits of omega-3 supplementation in reducing cortisol elevation.

Researchers in Japan (Hamazaki, *Biofactors,* 2000) showed decreased norepinephrine concentration (31 percent less) in students given 1.5 grams of DHA (one of the two key fatty acids in fish, the other is EPA) during exam week. They also showed a marked reduction in measures of hostility (72 percent less) in students on EPA supplementation compared to controls, when faced with the stress from final exams. (Norepinephrine, the acute stress hormone of the autonomic nervous system and the midbrain, will eventually lead to higher cortisol levels when chronically elevated.)

All these studies have the same conclusion: if enough of the right fats are eaten, the brain will not respond excessively to stress. The fats in the diet matter in terms of brain health and adaptation since they are incorporated right into the brain itself. This was also the opinion of other researchers including Lanfranco (*Journal of Clinical Endocrinology and Metabolism,* 2004) who found that essential fatty acid administration inhibits cortisol production through a mechanism in the brain itself, not in the pituitary or the adrenal gland. Another study went even further and showed that in mice who have brain lesions similar to Alzheimer's disease, use of essential fatty acids reduced damage to the hippocampus during stress and prevented the development of Alzheimer's-like brain lesions.

In addition to eating fatty fish such as wild salmon, to control cortisol levels it is helpful to supplement with EPA-DHA capsules on days when fish is not consumed. A reasonable dose for cortisol balance and adaptation is 1000–1200 mg of EPA and at least half as much DHA. Most supplements have between 160 and 320 mg of EPA per capsule. If you have any bleeding problems or use anticoagulants, fish-oil use needs to be supervised by a physician. Some people cannot tolerate fish oils without digestive upset. It is important to use a good antioxidant supplement if high-dose fish oil is used to prevent oxidative stress from the oils.

Linoleic Acid Supplementation

A study by Bruder (*Hormone Metabolism Research* 2006), found a connection between gamma linoleic acid (primrose, borage, and black currant seed oils) and reduction of cortisol production. An oxidized derivative of linoleic acid (EKODE) reduced cortisol production by 25 percent in adrenal cells. It also increased DHEA production, the other main adrenal hormone that reduces the destructive effect of cortisol by promoting tissue repair. It is thought that these fatty acids are oxidized in the liver and form compounds that modulate adrenal steroidogenesis, changing the amounts of cortisol and DHEA the adrenal gland produces.

Supplementing the diet with one of these oils is the easiest way to obtain the key omega 6 fatty acid, DGLA. Although this study looked at a synthetic derivative of these oils, I have observed improvement in my patients with symptoms such as premenstrual tension and anxiety with the use of evening primrose, borage, and black currant seed oils.

Phosphatidylserine

Phosphatidylserine (PS) is a major component of cell membranes and may restore sensitivity to cortisol receptors in the midbrain, hypothalamus, and pituitary to improve the feedback loop when cortisol levels are elevated. This is particularly important since long-term elevation of cortisol can damage the cells in the hippocampus that regulate cortisol secretion, disrupting the normal feedback control over production of this hormone.

I have used phosphatidylserine with my patients to help dampen excess cortisol production, improve memory, and treat depression. I often have them use it at night if there are symptoms of insomnia, anxiety, and memory loss. If tests reveal elevated cortisol at other times of the day, I use the PS at those times. Elevated nighttime cortisol occurs with breakdown of the feedback to the midbrain and is strongly associated with depression, anxiety, and insomnia.

Phosphatidylserine was first isolated in 1943 and has been extensively studied in over three thousand papers. It contains both fatty acids like DHA, an omega 3 essential fatty acid, and amino acids. It is vital to the function of brain cells and other cells throughout the body. Dietary sources of PS are organ meats, chicken skin, fatty fish, and meats. The average daily intake in Western diets is 130 mg; however a low fat diet provides even less. In the 1980s, the average intake was 250 mg. Modern food production of fats and oils decreases all the natural phospholipids in our diets, including phosphatidylserine.

Phosphatidylserine, (like phosphatidylcholine found in lecithin), are phospholipids that are incorporated into cell membranes, especially in the brain. In a study of healthy men given 800 mg of PS, the cortisol response to physical stress was blunted. Even as little as 75 mg of PS has shown reduction of cortisol response to physical stress. In a 2004 double-blind study of healthy men and women, PS (400 mg per day) compared to placebo significantly blunted cortisol response to psychological stress (Trier Social Stress Scale).

Phosphatidylserine improves communication between cells in the brain by increasing the number of membrane receptor sites for receiving messages. Phosphatidylserine modulates the fluidity of cell membranes, essential to the brain cells' ability to send and receive chemical communication.

Stress increases the demand for phosphatidylserine. Supplementing with PS has been shown to reduce exercise-induced stress by blunting the increase of cortisol after intense exercise. Studies have found that PS enhances mood and relaxation in stressful situations and increases dopamine production, helping with depression. It enhances metabolism of glucose in the brain, improving neurotransmitter function. It increases the synthesis of acetycholine, needed for memory, leading the FDA to state that it may reduce the risk of cognitive dysfunction in the elderly. PS has also been recommended for treating ADD and ADHD in children and adults. (Many of the studies with the strongest results for treating cognitive decline, even in Alzheimer's disease, were based on animal-derived PS from bovine brain tissue, which is no longer in use because of mad cow disease. The jury is still out on soy-based PS for these severe problems.)

The adaptogen effect of phosphatidylserine appears to be multifocal, including enhanced neurotransmitter release, which can moderate cortisol levels. By blunting the excess release of cortisol and sensitizing the feedback loop to the midbrain, there is less risk for allostatic load. Most supplements of phosphatidylserine are soy derived with a typical dose of 100 mg up to three times per day. If insomnia is an issue, one of the doses should be one hour before sleep.

Vitamin D

Vitamin D has emerged recently as a nutritional superstar. Among its many proven benefits are improving bone density and preventing osteoporosis, reducing the risk for prostate, colon, and breast cancer, improving immunity to viral infections, reducing the risk of heart disease and diabetes, and reducing the incidence of autoimmune diseases including multiple sclerosis and systemic lupus erythematosis. It is this last finding regarding reduction of autoimmune processes that makes vitamin D important in the world of adaptogens.

A telling study on vitamin D and inflammation looked at sixty-nine healthy women and measured vitamin D levels in the blood (25 OH vitamin D3). The women with the highest level of vitamin D had the lowest markers of inflammation including TNF alpha, a key lymphokine indicating immune activation. Women with regular UVB sun exposure had serum 25(OH) D concentrations that were significantly higher and parathyroid hormone concentrations that were significantly lower than women without regular UVB exposure.

Vitamin D deficiency affects between 30 percent and 50 percent of the general population. This epidemic is a result of many factors. Vitamin D gets activated from sunlight and UVB rays. As people age, the skin is less adept at converting precursors into vitamin D. In addition, the use of sunscreen and the presence of air pollution block vitamin D activation. Especially in children, reduction in outdoor time has contributed to this alarming increase in vitamin D deficiency. Vitamin D is formed in the skin from 7-dehydrocholesterol and then converted in the liver and kidney to the active form. Adequate sunlight would theoretically provide 90 percent of the needed amount of about 10,000 IU per day. However studies show that is clearly not happening. Possibly another factor in this epidemic of low vitamin D levels is the overuse of statin drugs, which lower cholesterol, the precursor of vitamin D in the skin.

Low vitamin D levels appear to be a major risk factor for cardiovascular disease. Low levels lead to high renin levels and hypertension, inflammation, insulin resistance, and increased risk of diabetes. Low vitamin D has also been linked to unexplained muscle pain, fatigue, poor resistance to infections, and a variety of autoimmune conditions. Vitamin

D supplementation, which achieves ideal blood levels, could lead to lower cortisol requirements by reducing inflammation and immune system problems. Normal blood levels of 25 OH vitamin D3 are from 30–100 ng/ml (nanograms per milliliter) with ideal levels between 40 and 80 ng/ml. Many of my patients are at the lower end of normal or even below 30 ng/ml, despite living in one of the sunniest climates in the United States.

In the past, normal vitamin D blood levels were thought to be lower. However, after studying groups in tropical areas, like Central American natives, it was realized that blood levels should be significantly higher and might reduce the incidence of multiple sclerosis, a disease with a greater incidence the father north one lives. It was also noted that vitamin D is needed to reduce the number of inflammatory cells in the brain of MS patients. In a study of 180,000 women, those who took 400 IU of vitamin D were 40 percent less likely to develop multiple sclerosis. These findings led researchers to suggest that maintaining higher levels of vitamin D could influence the occurrence of MS and other autoimmune conditions.

Lupus is another example of how low vitamin D possibly contributes to autoimmunity and inflammation. Several reports have shown that inadequate levels of vitamin D are frequently found in lupus patients, contributing to this inflammatory condition. In other studies in obese patients, vitamin D supplementation significantly improved markers of inflammation reducing the risk of cardiovascular disease.

In the past, the recommended doses of vitamin D supplementation were also too low and not based on good science since there was a lack of understanding of the crucial nature of this vitamin. It was assumed that sunlight would be enough and if any extra D was needed a teaspoon of cod liver oil (with about 400 IU) was adequate. Current research supports using doses of up to 5000 IU to achieve a blood level of 40 ng/ml, the minimum found to reduce inflammation and help prevent heart disease, cancer, hypertension and other major disease.

If signs of deficiency exist, I recommend at least 2000 IU of vitamin D3 in an oil-based form, though many patients need quite a bit more to achieve ideal blood levels. Higher doses require monitoring with blood tests to prevent toxicity since vitamin D is fat soluble and can cause problems with calcium metabolism and parathyroid secretion while increasing the risk of kidney stones. It should be used cautiously in anyone with high blood calcium levels or a history of kidney stones.

Botanical Adaptogens

Adaptogens, a term first proposed by Soviet researchers in the 1950s, are a group of natural substances including herbs and vitamins that improve responsiveness to stress and prevent allostatic load. The original research from the Soviets was focused on surviving extreme physical stress. However, my experience with patients under emotional stress as well as physical stress who become maladapted has demonstrated that these botanicals are helpful not only in the Gulags of Siberia, but in daily life.

Most adaptogens work through modification of cortisol production, leading to enhanced immune function, stress responsiveness, and the ability to recover from physical and emotional challenges. Though the exact mechanism of action for these herbs has not been identified, it is thought that they restore hypothalamic and midbrain sensitivity to modify cortisol production. Research has also shown that adaptogens affect tolerance for stress through their phytonutrient (flavonoids, lignans, carotenoids) content, acting as antioxidants and membrane stabilizers. They have demonstrated immune-regulatory and blood sugar stabilizing effects, further leading to reduced cortisol response.

Adaptogens reduce an excessive immediate fight-or-flight response and elevated epinephrine and norepinephrine levels, as well as reducing allostatic load and adrenal exhaustion. They reduce symptoms of fatigue by making cellular energy production more efficient and reducing lactic acid buildup (from inefficient anaerobic metabolism). Adaptogens also improve the homeostatic mechanism, overcoming allostatic load and reestablishing allostasis.

Another benefit described for adaptogens is a normalization effect. For example, if one person has elevated blood pressure as a result of stress, while another experiences blood pressure drops when stressed, adaptogens through improvement of the midbrain and the hypothalamic pituitary axis normalize blood pressure response either raising or lowering it as required. Adaptogens can reduce excessive host defense reactions, decreasing the damaging effect of allostatic load, while at the same time allowing for an appropriate response to stress.

Breakdown of the cortisol feedback control mechanism during long-term stress occurs because of neuro-potentiation of the amygdala, decreased sensitivity in the hippocampus, and increased locus coeruleus production of epinephrine from CRH stimulation. The hypothalamus is affected by all these changes. In some cases this will lead to a lack of responsiveness in the midbrain to appropriately stimulate cortisol release when in stressful situations. This is the "adrenal exhaustion" phase mistakenly thought by many as a problem with the adrenal gland itself. Since part of the effect of adaptogens is thought to occur at the hypothalamic level, it is possible that their impact can also be on the midbrain, resetting its control over cortisol production. The botanical adaptogens that I use the most in my practice include Siberian ginseng, Chinese (Panax) ginseng, ashwagandha, rhodiola rosea, ginkgo biloba, and cordyceps sinensis.

It is imperative that these botanicals be used with medical supervision if there is any concern about a medical condition or any blood-thinning medications are used. Each of these herbs might affect any one individual in a negative manner if the person's current state of the HPA axis does not call for the specific effect of the adaptogen. These are powerful herbs with multiple effects and should be treated with respect.

Siberian Ginseng

One of the most widely studied adaptogens is Siberian ginseng (*eleutherococcus senticosus*). Russian scientists in the 1950s discovered that this herb, distinct from Chinese or Korean ginseng (Panax ginseng), had powerful adaptogenic properties. Clinical studies in over 2100 healthy human subjects given Siberian ginseng as a supplement showed an increased ability to adapt to adverse physical conditions as well as improved mental performance and enhanced quality of work under stressful conditions. It has shown strong antioxidant effects and the ability to protect nerve and heart cells from damage.

Siberian ginseng has six compounds that are antioxidants, four with anticancer activity, three that lower cholesterol, two that stimulate the immune system, and one that modulates insulin levels. Studies on Siberian ginseng (over a thousand have been done, most in Russia and other countries previously in the Soviet bloc) showed improved adaptation in several areas.

Table 1 Soviet studies on Siberian ginseng and Effects on Adaptation

- A 40 percent decrease in high blood pressure and a 30 percent decrease in total reported symptoms in auto factory workers
- A 30 percent reduction in the incidence of influenza in long-distance truck drivers
- Improved stamina and recovery in Soviet Olympic athletes
- A 50 percent decrease in immune suppression from chemotherapy in patients with gastric cancer
- Increased endurance in Soviet cosmonauts during long-duration space flights

Siberian ginseng appears to improve hypothalamic receptor sensitivity, leading to reduced abnormal cortisol production, less immune suppression, lower blood pressure, and improved glucose metabolism. It acted as a true adaptogen in studies demonstrating increased cortisol output below a stress threshold and decreased output above a stress threshold, enhancing the physiologic response to mild stress and modulating the response to extreme stress. It prevents some of the immune suppression seen with elevated cortisol. Studies have shown that Siberian ginseng normalizes blood sugar through stimulating the release of glycogen stored in muscles for immediate energy, reducing long-term elevation of glucose and insulin resistance and reducing catabolic (muscle-wasting) effects on muscle and endurance.

I generally recommend the use of a combination of adaptogens to improve adaptation. The dose of Siberian ginseng in most formulations is 200 mg containing 0.8 percent eleutheroids E and B. The active compounds for most adaptogens have been identified and are usually listed as a percentage of total ingredients. For example, the eleutheroids are the active compounds in Siberian ginseng and should comprise at least 0.8 percent of total compounds.

Panax Ginseng

The other ginseng often used, Asian (also called Korean) or Panax ginseng has different active compounds (ginsenosides) than Siberian ginseng. Panax ginseng has a long history of use in Chinese medicine, employed as a tonic to improve energy and adaptation. It appears to improve the feedback loop of the hypothalamic-pituitary-adrenal axis. In one study reported by Le Gal (*Phytotherapy Research* 1996) the use of 80 mg of Panax ginseng per day in addition to a multivitamin was associated with a significant improvement in energy levels in most participants in the study.

Panax ginseng has a variety of actions on the adrenal gland and HPA axis. In animals, it has been shown to increase the size of adrenal cells, enhancing activity. It can increase HPA sensitivity to cortisol through effects on the hypothalamus. Certain ginsenosides have shown buffering ability to reduce an exaggerated adrenal stress response. In the brain, ginseng stimulates ACTH and the cortisol response to acute stress but also demonstrates improved negative feedback and greater sensitivity of the brain to circulating levels of cortisol, reducing allostatic load. It can up-regulate the HPA, reduce fatigue, and is especially useful in the later stages of HPA underfunctioning. Typical doses range from 100 mg to 400 mg with 8 percent ginsenosides.

Ashwagandha

Ashwagandha (*withania somnifera*) is another invaluable adaptogen. It has been used for centuries in Indian Ayurvedic medicine. Studies show that ashwagandha improves adaptation to both physical and emotional stress. Animals pretreated with this adaptogen and exposed to stressful conditions did not have as much adrenal hypertrophy, blood sugar elevation, or cortisol depletion as untreated animals. Ashwagandha also has anabolic activity (increasing androgens needed for tissue repair such as DHEA), and normalizes inflammatory prostaglandins. It also reduces catecholamine (epinephrine) production and normalizes blood sugar and cholesterol levels.

People treated with ashwagandha report feeling less anxious in stressful situations. It appears to enhance GABA levels and in animal models has a neuorestorative effect in Parkinson's and Alzheimer's disease. In addition, it demonstrates significant immune-enhancing effects as well as anti-inflammatory properties. Other stress-modifying-effects include reduction of the incidence of peptic ulcers and improvement of thyroid function. Typical dosages of ashwaganda are 200 mg containing 5 percent withanolides.

Rhodiola Rosea

Rhodiola rosea (also called Arctic root) is native to high mountainous areas of Asia and Eastern Europe. It is another herb that the Soviets studied extensively, finding that it enhanced work performance and resistance to stress. I have found it is one of the most clinically useful adaptogens, especially when combined with phosphatidylserine, which improves the midbrain's response to stress.

Rhodiola appears to affect neurotransmitters including dopamine, serotonin, catecholamines, and beta-endorphins. It is also cardio-protective, maintaining higher levels of cAMP (an energy-producing enzyme) in the heart muscle. It reduces catecholamine stimulation of cardiac tissue leading to less arrhythmia. It is often useful in the person that is easily overstimulated and is wired and tired. It also stimulates immune function while reducing stress-induced beta-endorphin production. (Beta-endorphin and ACTH are both produced in the pituitary as a response to stress.) Rhodiola has been studied extensively for more than thirty-five years. In a study of work-fatigued physicians, rhodiola produced an improvement in cognitive function and performance. The dose is about 200 mg containing at least 1 percent salidrosides.

Ginkgo Biloba

Ginkgo biloba is a well-researched herb that has strong adaptogenic properties. It reduces elevated cortisol levels and can increase ACTH levels. Ginkgo has been shown to reduce stress-induced learning impairment in rats and potentially to reduce stress-induced cognitive dysfunction in humans. It increases acetylcholine synthesis and the turnover of norepinephrine.

Ginkgo has been shown to reverse age-related losses of adrenergic receptors in the neocortical area of the brain. It increases uptake of choline in the hippocampus and could have an anticonvulsant effect. Thirteen studies with a combined 936 patients supported the use of ginkgo in dementia and demonstrated slowing of clinical deterioration and improvement of cognitive function.

Ginkgo protects mitochondria from oxidative damage and has potent antioxidant effects that are protective of brain tissue. Ginkgo has been shown to increase blood flow in the central nervous system. It has a mild anticoagulant effect inhibiting platelet aggregation that improves the general circulation. Ginkgo can improve cognitive function and possibly slow degenerative disease of the brain. Supplements should contain at least 120 mg with 24 percent of the active ingredient, ginkgo flavonglycosides. Caution should be used if surgery is imminent or blood-thinning medications are combined with ginkgo.

Cordyceps

Another potent adaptogen, especially useful with "adrenal fatigue," is cordyceps sinensis, a medicinal mushroom that is one of the most valued therapies in Chinese medicine. Wild cordyceps is a rare, blade-shaped fungus found at high altitudes in China and Tibet. Chinese scientists have been able to produce a water-soluble extract of the mycelial component of the fungus that contains the active ingredients cordycepic acid and adenosine.

Cordyceps has been used in traditional Chinese medicine to support vitality, improve kidney and lung function, and enhance libido. It has been shown to have beneficial effects on immune function as well as normalizing glucose metabolism. As an adaptogen, cordyceps has been shown to have substantial effects on adrenal function.

Studies have shown that the hot water extract of cordyceps improves endurance of mice in response to physical stress, inhibits cholesterol elevation, and inhibits enlargement of the adrenal gland. (The size of the adrenal gland is often used as a measure of stress effects because chronic allostatic load typically increases the size of the adrenal gland as the body attempts to react to the stressful situation.) Another study showed adrenal cells from rats increased their ability to secrete cortisol when stimulated with cordyceps in a manner differing from stimulation by ACTH.

Cordyceps is most useful when fatigue and anxiety are significant symptoms. In human studies, cordyceps improved fatigue, cold intolerance, and cognitive function in elderly people. It has been shown to improve stress tolerance and endurance in animal studies. Cordyceps has also demonstrated an ability to improve respiratory function in patients with COPD (emphysema) and increase energy levels in patients with heart failure. It has many effects on the immune system, increasing T-cell activity, promoting natural killer-cell function, protecting against the effects of radiation therapy, and reducing inflammation in autoimmune states. Like other medicinal mushrooms, cordyceps has shown apoptotic (cell death) effects in cancer-cell lines including leukemia and colon and liver cancer. A typical adaptogenic dose to help with cortisol control is 400 mg of the hot-water extract standardized to contain 8 percent cordycepic acid and 0.25 percent adenosine, taken twice daily.

Licorice

Another approach to controlling cortisol production is the use of licorice extracts (carbenoxolone) to inhibit the conversion of cortisone to cortisol by adipocytes. These extracts can block the 11HSD1 enzymes needed to convert inactive cortisone to cortisol in fat cells. It is possible that using small amounts of licorice-root extracts (not Red Vines or other licorice candies) can slow down the production of cortisol.

One other effect of licorice is mimicking the physiologic effects of aldosterone to raise blood pressure. This can be most helpful in people who are fatigued and have low blood pressure but can be a problem in hypertensives. Careful monitoring and change in dose as needed can be required with the use of licorice extracts.

Table 2: Typical Adaptogen Dosages

- Panax ginseng 200 mg to 400 mg with 8 percent ginsenosides
- Eleuthorococcus 200 mg containing 0.8 percent eleutheroids E and B
- Ashwaganda (withonia somnifera) 200 mg containing 5 percent withanolides
- Rhodiola rosea 200 mg containing at least 1 percent salidrosides
- Ginkgo biloba 120 mg with 24 percent ginkgo flavonglycosides
- Codyceps sinensis 400 mg of hot-water extract containing 8 percent cordycepic acid and 0.25 percent adenosine, taken twice daily

Nutrient Adaptogens

I'm using the term *nutrient adaptogens* to describe vitamins, minerals, fatty acids, and sterols that have been shown to improve allostasis and the body's response to stress. Before the availability in my practice of many of the botanicals listed above, I relied on vitamins such as pantothenic acid (B5) and vitamin C to modify cortisol function. Following are the most useful of these nutritional adaptogens.

Most of the research on vitamin C has been to evaluate the antioxidant, immune-enhancing, and tissue-repairing properties of this critical vitamin. However it also has a strong effect on cortisol production. I have found in my practice that high dose vitamin C mimics the effect of cortisol, reducing inflammation and allergies and thereby reducing the need for cortisol production. For example, a study by Carrillo of marathon runners who took 1500 mg of vitamin C a day for one week before a race found significantly lower post-race cortisol levels than those given 500 mg or a placebo.

A study on the effect of vitamin C on cortisol levels from elevated psychological stress (Trier Social Stress Test, which measures response to mental arithmetic and mock job interviews) demonstrated lower subjective stress levels, cortisol levels, and blood pressure in individuals who took 3000 mg of vitamin C compared to placebo. The minimum dose of vitamin C needed for an adaptogenic response is 1000 mg per day, preferably in the form of a buffered ascorbate, not ascorbic acid.

Another old standby in my practice is pantothenic acid, or vitamin B5. It is found in many foods including eggs, yeast, meat, poultry, and whole grains, yet despite its widespread availability, many of my patients respond to supplementation. Deficiency of B5 compromises adrenal function, while studies have shown that B5 can down-regulate hypersecretion of cortisol secondary to high-stress conditions. Fatigue and intolerance to stress can be a sign of B5 deficiency.

B vitamins have long been known to help with stress. The most research has been done on pyridoxine or vitamin B6. Deficiency of B6 leads to increased sympathetic nervous system outflow and even hypertension. In animal studies, supplementing with B6 has reduced the levels of epinephrine as well as blunting the cortisol response. Deficiency of B6 also leads to reduced production of GABA and serotonin, neurotransmitters that reduce anxiety and depression.

In a study of bereavement-induced psychological stress, low B6 levels worsened the maladapted state. Twenty-five years ago, pyridoxine was called the "anti-stress factor" because it was shown to prevent increased tissue sensitivity to cortisol. It appears that B6 decreases glucocorticoid-mediated protein induction, down-regulating the tissue response to cortisol, while severe pyridoxine deficiency strongly up-regulates cellular response to cortisol.

Supplementing with high-dose B6 (up to 200 mg per day) could be required to see a marked reduction in stress-hormone responsiveness. The active form of B6, pyridoxal-5-phosphate, is now available, and doses of 50–100 mg daily might be enough to achieve the same effect. Studies done as early as the 1970s have shown clinical improvement with B6 in depression and stress reactions through diminishing sympathetic nervous system overactivity and decreasing cortisol production evoked by stress.

A word of caution on the use of high dose B vitamins is warranted. They should be used under the supervision of an experienced physician since high dose B6 has been associated with peripheral nerve problems when used without other B vitamins. I always have patients use 1000 micrograms of B12 as well as 1 mg of folic acid and a well-balanced B complex when taking B6 above 50 mg a day. B12 and folic acid have their own adaptogenic effects and should be part of a well-rounded nutritional approach to maladaptation.

Table 3: Adaptogenic Nutrients

- B6 up to 200 mg per day or P-5P at 100 mg per day
- B5 (pantothenic acid) 100–500 mg per day
- B complex 50 mg per day
- B12 500–1000 mcg per day in a sublingual tablet
- Vitamin C 1000 mg per day
- Phosphatidylserine 200–400 mg per day
- Multivitamin and mineral (preferably from a reputable vitamin company that has more than the RDA minimums and contains at least 400 mcg of folic acid)

Chapter Eight

The Curious Cases of Gluten and Candida

The cultivation of wheat and other grains was a watershed moment in human evolution, providing a stable and nutritious food source and moving our early ancestors from hunter-gatherers to a society able to develop cities and commerce. Wheat is believed to have originated in southwestern Asia; some of the earliest remains of the crop have been found in Syria, Jordan, and Turkey. Primitive relatives of present day wheat have been discovered in excavations in eastern Iraq dating back nine thousand years. Other archeological findings show that wheat was grown in the Nile Valley about 5000 BC, as well as in India, China, and even England at about the same time. Despite this illustrious history, wheat and other grains are a common trigger of maladaptation and allostatic load, linked to conditions such as celiac disease, osteoporosis, headaches, joint pain, and digestive inflammation.

When I was growing up in New York, one of my family jobs was to go to the neighborhood bakery to buy a loaf of freshly baked rye bread before dinner. By the time I got home, I had consumed four or five slices, cutting into my appetite much to the chagrin of my mother. That same degree of craving is not uncommon in my adult patients, as wheat is one of the most addictive of all foods. Wheat uniquely contains exorphins, a substance similar to endorphins, the pain-relieving and mood-elevating chemicals made by the brain. After digestion of a slice of bread or serving of pasta, the exorphins from wheat go to the same brain receptors as endorphins, explaining the addictive nature of this food.

It doesn't make much sense that a food that was integral to human evolution has caused so many people health problems. However, like many things in life, too much of a good thing has become a problem for some people. Sensitivity to gluten (the protein in wheat) is widespread in the Untied States, especially in people of Northern European extraction (Scandinavian, English, Irish, and German).

Gluten is found in wheat, barley, rye, malt, triticale, spelt, and kamut. It is found in the greatest amount in wheat and rye. There is some controversy about whether the protein in oats triggers the same response as glutens because it is a different branch of the Grass family of foods (figure 1) and contains avenin, not gluten protein. However, some of the oats commercially available can be contaminated with wheat and other grains and generally should be avoided. If pure oats can be obtained, 98 percent of celiac patients can use them without triggering inflammation. Hidden sources of gluten include many processed foods such as cold cuts and deli meats, frozen vegetables, soups, salad dressings, and soy sauce. Gluten is composed of gliadin and glutenin proteins.

Individuals vary in their response to gluten proteins. On one end of the continuum is simple gluten intolerance (also called nonceliac gluten intolerance) with symptoms of fatigue, headaches, digestive bloating, flatulence, diarrhea, weight gain, skin problems, depression, and joint or muscle pain. It is estimated that one in ten Americans could have gluten intolerance or wheat allergy. On the other end of the continuum is the more serious celiac disease, a less common problem with an incidence of 1 in every 133 Americans.

Table 1: Incidence of Gluten Intolerance and Celiac Disease

- 1 in 133 asymptomatic healthy Americans have celiac disease
- 1 in 11 with a family member with celiac disease
- 1 in 30 adults with digestive complaints have celiac
- 1 in 8 people with Northern European heritage have celiac
- 30 million Americans have gluten sensitivity
- 3 million Americans have been diagnosed with celiac disease
- 19 out of 20 cases go undetected

Grain Families

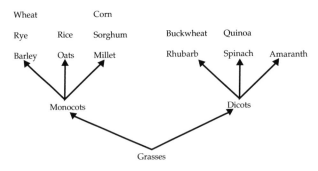

The Grain Families
From Celiac Disease: A Hidden Epidemic
By Peter H.R. Green, M.D. and Rory Jones

In celiac disease, gluten protein causes the destruction of the intestinal villa (fingerlike protrusions that provide most of the surface area for nutrient absorption) in the small intestine from exposure to the gluten protein in grains. It takes less than 1 gram per day of gliadin (less than 2 percent of an ounce) to cause an inflammatory response. This leads to malabsorption, weight loss, and severe fatigue and is associated with osteoporosis, autoimmunity, arthritis, and other systemic problems. One quarter of patients with celiac disease have a chronic skin condition known as dermatitis herpetiformis, which can include intense itching and blisters. Other conditions seen in celiac disease are listed in table 2.

Table 2: Conditions Associated with Celiac Disease

- Diabetes
- Obesity
- Depression
- Neuropathy
- Osteoporosis
- Thyroid disease
- Sjogren's syndrome
- Rheumatoid arthritis
- Autoimmune liver disease

The diagnosis of celiac disease is best made through an intestinal biopsy that demonstrates changes in the wall of the intestine including inflammation and atrophy. The only treatment for celiac disease is life-long avoidance of all gluten sources. It can be life saving to make this diagnosis. Nonceliac gluten intolerance does not involve any organ damage.

A minority of patients with celiac disease will have obvious symptoms: weight loss, diarrhea, cramping, and appearing ill. The more common presentation involves symptoms outside the gastrointestinal tract: neurological, endocrine, psychiatric, and rheumatologic. Malabsorption can lead to deficiencies in fat-soluble vitamins, including vitamin A needed for vision, skin, and reproductive function; vitamin D needed for bones, prevention of breast, ovarian, and prostate cancer, and normal immune function; vitamin E needed for heart health, antioxidant function, and detoxification; and vitamin K needed for blood clotting and strong bones. In addition, minerals such as calcium and iron can be deficient in celiac disease. This can lead to anemia and osteoporosis.

Fatigue and depression are common problems in both celiac and nonceliac gluten intolerance. Fatigue can be caused by a combination of malabsorption of nutrients, especially B vitamins, inflammation in the gut, iron deficiency, and anemia and autoimmunity affecting thyroid function. Depression is most likely a result of deficiency of fatty acids, such as EPA-DHA, which are needed for brain function, and lack of B12 and other B vitamins. Many times I have seen patients with gluten problems who were treated with antidepressants when they simply needed to change their diets.

Table 3: Nutrient Malabsorption in Celiac Disease

- Essential fatty acids, omega-3 and omega-6
- Iron, zinc, calcium, and magnesium
- Selenium
- Water soluble vitamins: B1, B6, B12, folic acid
- Fat soluble vitamins: A, D, E, K

Symptoms found with gluten intolerance are also often mistakenly attributed to other conditions. In addition to depression and fatigue, obesity, food cravings, diarrhea, constipation, lethargy and lack of interest in life, poor concentration, back pain, muscle cramps, and joint pain are commonly seen. It is not hard to imagine each of these complaints being treated with medications rather than identifying their underlying cause. Even in my practice, I have been fooled several times into thinking gluten intolerance was not the trigger for certain symptoms (table 4). However, by keeping an open mind regarding the varied presentations of gluten problems, eventually a diagnosis can be made. It has been estimated that on average it can take as long as nine years between the onset of symptoms and proper diagnosis of celiac disease or gluten intolerance.

Table 4: Common Symptoms of Gluten Intolerance

- Abdominal cramps, bloating, gas
- Diarrhea or constipation
- Poor concentration, brain fog
- Irritability and unpredictable moods
- Weight gain, obesity
- Long-standing fatigue
- Food craving especially for starches and sweets
- Depression

- Lethargy, lack of interest and motivation
- Joint pain, muscle cramps, muscle pain, back or neck pain
- Unexplained elevation of liver enzymes on blood tests
- Neuropathy

I have also found that in wheat allergy even without gluten intolerance, depression, fatigue, and anxiety are common symptoms. Many times in skin testing patients for food allergies with the provocative-neutralization technique, I have seen mood changes and problems with concentration, which resolve once this food is removed from the diet. The most common food that contributes to depression and cognitive issues is wheat. Avoidance and challenge as described in Chapter 4 is the best method to confirm a wheat allergy if appropriate skin testing is not available.

Diagnosis of these conditions can be difficult. Genetic markers found on cell surfaces through blood tests (HLA, DQ2, and DQ8) can be useful but often are not conclusive. Blood antibody tests for celiac disease (antigliadin antibodies including IgA endomysial antibodies, IgA tissue transglutaminase antibodies, and IgG tissue transglutaminase antibodies) are only positive in celiac disease and are often negative in gluten intolerance. Salivary IgA antigliadin antibodies can be a good screen but still present false negatives and false positives. The best way to identify gluten intolerance is avoidance of these foods for several months. If gluten is a significant trigger for allostatic load, many symptoms will improve within three months, though some problems might take as long as six months to resolve. If you are concerned that celiac disease is present, you should consult a gastroenterologist immediately for biopsy of the small intestine, which is more accurate while still ingesting gluten foods.

European physicians are much more aware of the problems that gluten can trigger than most physicians in the United States. We were on vacation in Ireland several years ago, and I was amazed to find that at a restaurant run by the national park service in Killarney Lakes National Park, there was a gluten-free section in the cafeteria. The Irish are particularly susceptible to this problem and have made great strides in making gluten-free foods available. Fortunately gluten-free grains and foods have recently become much more available in the United States.

Wheat allergy and gluten intolerance are different, though overlapping conditions. Strictly speaking, wheat allergy is a reaction to the albumin or globulin protein in wheat and not the glutens. Skin testing or blood-antibody tests can identify wheat allergy with different testing needed for gluten intolerance. Even in cases without the intestinal pathology of celiac disease (also called nontropical sprue), gluten intolerance causes some inflammation in the gut wall while food allergy to wheat might not involve the digestive track. This is a confusing area for my patients who had negative skin tests to wheat but still benefit greatly from gluten avoidance. Whether gluten intolerant, wheat allergic, or suffering from celiac disease, the result of eating wheat and other gluten grains is a dramatic increase in cortisol production to counteract the inflammatory changes induced by these conditions. To regain adaptation, it is critical to identify these problems and make the appropriate dietary changes to reduce cortisol and allostatic load.

Wheat-free (Weigh Less)

In the early 1990s I started an experiment to see if my patients could lose weight simply by eliminating gluten containing foods. They stopped eating all breads, muffins, baked goods, and pizza as well as cereals with wheat, rye, barley, and oats but did not cut their caloric content in other ways. We devised recipes for nongluten grains, though there were few good alternatives available then as compared to now. (When looking to see if a food is wheat free, remember wheat can be listed as durum, enriched, wheat germ, bulgur, couscous, triticale, orzo, or semolina.)

Almost every patient lost weight effortlessly if they stayed on strict gluten avoidance. They also noted improved energy, less muscle and joint pain, fewer headaches, better digestive function, and most surprisingly better moods and less anxiety. They reduced markers of inflammation and allostatic load and maladaptation. Many of them brought their cortisol levels back to an adapted state.

Alternatives to gluten are widely available. Though gluten is the material that causes grain to be sticky, yielding breads and baked products that are so satisfying, the new gluten-free products such as brown rice pastas can be quite good. Products made from rice, millet, buckwheat, amaranth, quinoa, potato, tapioca, and arrowroot provide a rich alternative to wheat and other gluten grains. For example, tapioca bagels are available through several Internet sources. Grain-free starches that are excellent sources of fiber and nutrients include yams, sweet potatoes, parsnips, winter squash, and other root vegetables.

Even if good alternatives to gluten exist, it is still wise to remember that refined grains should not be a large part of the diet. Eating refined grains including oats and wheat will increase caloric intake of other foods if eaten early in the day. In a study of obese children, Children's Hospital in Boston found that after a meal of instant oatmeal as compared to a vegetable omelet and fruit, children consumed 81 percent more calories throughout the day.

In another study of overweight adults performed in Italy, a high-carbohydrate meal activated the HPA axis and cortisol production to a much greater degree than a high-protein meal.

Combining gluten avoidance with the other aspects of the Adaptation Diet including limiting total grain intake, especially refined grains, makes weight loss even easier. For those people who are gluten intolerant, it is essential that these foods be removed from the diet to ensure reduction in stress and allostatic load. For anyone who wants to shed pounds and improve their tolerance for stress, a time-out for wheat and baked goods will pay off. At least three months is needed to have the desired effects. If gluten is not a major issue, it can be reintroduced at that time using a rotation diet. (See appendix section 5 for gluten-free recipes and diet plan.)

Gluten-Containing Foods—A Short List

- Beverages: coffee substitutes, malted drinks, beer, ale
- Baked goods: whole wheat, graham crackers, rolls, muffins, doughnuts, sweet rolls, pancakes, waffles, crackers, prepared bake mixes
- Cereals: wheat, barley, rye, some oats
- Animal protein: possible in deli meats, packaged cold cuts, chili con carne, croquettes, fish or meat patties, and loaves
- Thick liquids, condiments, and sauces: malt products, soups, chowders, soy sauce, bisques thickened with wheat

The Candida Connection

One of the most powerful regulators of adaptation is a healthy intestinal tract. Since the early 1980s when William Crook identified a common syndrome of yeast overgrowth in the digestive tract and the resulting increased inflammation, food allergies, and poor well-being, a controversy has raged about a lowly inhabitant of the gut, a yeastlike organism, *candida albicans.* Despite tremendous resistance from traditional medicine in recognizing this problem, my patients have benefited to an enormous degree from treating *candida* overgrowth syndrome. Let me explain why this is so controversial.

Within the first year of life, essentially all human digestive tracts are colonized with *candida albicans.* Unlike other beneficial inhabitants of the gut such as lactobacillus and bifidobacter, *candida* provides no benefit to the host. Since it is found in everyone, academic medicine has scoffed at the idea that it contributes to any problems other than yeast vaginitis in women, penile rashes in men, and thrush in the mouth. It is known to be a problem in the colonization of internal organs in immunosuppressed patients with AIDS or patients on medications that suppress the immune response. Except in those extreme circumstances, *candida* is not found in body cavities except in the digestive tract and the vaginal area in women.

However, even in patients who are not severely ill, *candida* can contribute to allostatic load. The digestive tract has the ability to be tolerant to *candida* if it is found in small amounts or if the immune system in the gut is operating in a normal fashion. Unfortunately, through the use of medications and poor diet, tolerance to *candida* can be lost. This frequently occurs from the excessive use of antibiotics for infections, acne, or other reasons. These medications reduce the amount of beneficial bacteria in the gut that produce lactic acid, which controls the proliferation of *candida* and other unwanted inhabitants of the gastrointestinal tract. *Candida* then overgrows, adhering to the wall in the large intestine, creating an excessive immune response to this fungal organism, sensitizing the body to other allergens.

Overgrowth of *candida* can even result from the ingestion of the antibiotics found in meats and poultry. Any use of prescription cortisone (Prednisone), some birth control pills, or most importantly, diets with excessive sweets and simple carbohydrates help *candida* prosper. *Candida* in the gut, like nutritional yeast in bread or wine, thrives in a high-sugar environment. White flour products including breads and other baked goods, processed sugars of any type, and even the natural sugars found in fruit juice or dried fruit can lead to more growth. Alcohol is an especially important trigger for yeast growth.

Candida is a constant irritant to the immune system, causing increased production of inflammatory cytokines, leading to bowel symptoms of bloating and gas, fatigue, aches and pains, and other markers of allostatic load. It appears to up-regulate the immune system so that there are greater sensitivities to molds, foods, and chemical substances. In addition, there is an increase in food allergy problems and worsening of the leaky-gut syndrome. In some women there will be an increased frequency of yeast vaginitis.

Testing for *candida* overgrowth is not straightforward since there is always some growth in the gut, and a normal immune system should react to *candida* skin testing. In my practice I use a quantitative stool culture to assess excess colonization. I skin test patients and look for a heightened skin wheal response. However, often the most useful diagnostic information is a history of antibiotic use leading to symptoms of yeast overgrowth. As in many other aspects of medicine, the ultimate diagnosis of *candida* overgrowth is the response to treatment.

Symptoms of *candida* overgrowth include fatigue, stamina problems, frequent infections, mood swings, allergies, and poor stress tolerance. I have listed below the key signs and symptoms for this problem.

Table 5: Signs and Symptoms of Candida Overgrowth

- Bloating of the abdomen, flatulence, poor digestive function
- Fatigue and stamina issues
- Mood swings, depression, irritability
- PMS, menstrual irregularity
- Recurrent yeast vaginitis, especially from use of antibiotics
- Frequent colds and flu
- Allergies to molds, foods
- Acute sense of smell and adverse reactions to chemicals such as paints, varnishes, car exhaust, gasoline, cleaning detergents
- Frequent or persistent antibiotic use
- Multiple pregnancies or high-dose birth control pills
- Use of steroid medications

Many times a vicious cycle of poor diet leading to more frequent infections and more prescriptions for antibiotics results in *candida* overgrowth. This then leads to more allergies, poor immune function, fatigue, and more infections. Another significant contributor to this cycle is elevated cortisol from other maladaptive causes. High cortisol and elevated blood sugar induce *candida* overgrowth. For example, it is well known that diabetics are much more prone to yeast infections and problems from *candida*. The consequence of overgrowth of *candida* is increased biochemical stress that then triggers even more cortisol production, and the cycle continues.

Though this seems like a dreadful situation, there are effective means to reduce *candida* overgrowth and bring tolerance back to the immune system. The first step is dietary. I have used the anti-yeast diet (see appendix section 6) in my practice for the past twenty years to reduce the stimulus for *candida* overgrowth. It is essentially the Adaptation Diet with a few minor changes. Simple carbohydrates, alcohol, and concentrated fruit sugars are the most important foods to avoid. Yeast growth is directly stimulated by these foods. The second concern is the total amount of carbohydrate consumed. I instruct my patients to avoid all gluten grains, starchy vegetables like white potatoes, fruit juice, and to reduce their overall intake of fruits for the first two months.

The third group of foods to avoid are those that contain molds and yeast. The concern with these foods is a cross sensitivity to food molds as well as to the *candida* overgrowth in the gut. Foods in this group include any hard cheese, aged cheese like blue cheese, vinegar, mushrooms, dried fruit, fruits such as melons and the skins of peaches and apricots. Yeast-containing foods such as bread and baked goods are to be strictly eliminated. Following the guidelines of the Adaptation Diet and making these few additional changes will help to control the yeast overgrowth. Usually three months on an anti-yeast diet will make a big difference in allostatic load.

Highlights of the Anti-Yeast Diet

- Adaptation Diet is the core diet
- Focus on vegetables, proteins, legumes
- Avoid all simple sugars including cane sugar, corn sweeteners, honey, molasses, fructose, and milk sugar in milk products
- No alcohol
- Condiments like ketchup and mustard have sugar added and should be avoided
- Avoid malt in cereals and other foods
- Processed and canned foods often contain sugar products
- Avoid all gluten grains (wheat, rye, barley); use only whole non-gluten grains
- Reduce the overall carbohydrate load
- Avoid breads and all yeast containing foods
- No aged or moldy foods including brick and aged cheeses, vinegar, mushrooms, dried fruits, melons
- Avoid leftovers if there is any chance of mold contamination

In addition to diet, good self-care is critical in managing *candida* overgrowth. Exercise, rest, and managing stress effectively will assist the immune system in increasing tolerance. Most important is the avoidance of antibiotics whenever possible. For most viral respiratory infections, antibiotics are not needed, though they are often prescribed. As an alternative, if there are no signs of a bacterial infection, botanical therapies could be employed including high dose vitamin C, echinacea, astragalus, maitake extracts, and lactoferrin as well as a variety of homeopathic compounds.

Probiotic therapy is very important in controlling yeast overgrowth, including high potency lactobacillus and bifidus combinations. Specific botanical therapies are also useful, including plant tannins, uva ursi, gentian, caprylic acid, oregano oil, berberine, colloidal silver, and undecyclic acid. In some cases antifungal medications such as Nystatin, Diflucan or Sporonox are needed. All these therapies have to be used under the direction of an experienced health care provider.

> Many of my patients have experienced profound improvements in their health after reducing *candida* overgrowth. Roberta, a mother of three children, was 37 years old when she consulted me for a long list of problems including fatigue, digestive bloating, muscle and joint pains, and most bothersome to her family, mood swings and severe premenstrual tension syndrome (PMS). She had allergies as a child and had received many courses of antibiotics for respiratory infections.
>
> Roberta suffered from frequent yeast vaginitis, often after taking antibiotics for her recurrent respiratory infections. In addition, her allergies were returning after a hiatus of fifteen years, and she became sensitive to perfumes and cleaning materials. In addition to fatigue, she had problems with her memory and mental focus.
>
> Roberta had intense cravings for sweets, breads, and other starches. Her *candida* testing revealed a very high level of growth in her digestive tract. I prescribed the anti-yeast diet (see appendix section 6), antifungal medications, probiotics and antifungal botanicals for her.
>
> Within a month Roberta was a new person. Although she struggled to stop eating desserts and breads, her bloating and aches and pains diminished. Her energy returned and even the PMS was greatly reduced. What amazed her the most was her mental clarity. Roberta felt she had emerged from a fog. As she was able to control her sugar cravings and maintained the anti-yeast diet over the next three months, Roberta's allergies greatly improved as well.

Though the diet needed to suppress *candida* overgrowth is restrictive, there are still many options, even on a restaurant menu. Order carefully, skip the cocktail and wine and the breads and desserts, and the rest is relatively easy. Order entrées without sauces, grilled, broiled or baked; and eat all the salads (skip the dressing) and vegetables you want. This diet is similar to the detoxification phase of the Adaptation Diet. Reducing yeast overgrowth for some of my patients was the most significant way to reduce their allostatic load and regain adaptation. If there is suspicion of *candida* overgrowth and it does not resolve from careful dietary management, consult with a physician familiar with this problem to determine what else should be done.

Chapter Nine
Conclusion

My clinical experience has taught me that food can have a great impact on the ability to adapt to stressful circumstances. These ideas have had such a significant effect on my patients that I wanted to share these insights with others. Increasing cortisol production and the stress response through the consumption of bad fats, allergic foods, and high-glycemic carbohydrates leads to greater vulnerability to the inevitable stress that accompanies our lives. It is my job as a physician to not only help people recover from illness, but to do everything possible to optimize well-being and reduce the likelihood of chronic disease. Modern research has demonstrated conclusively that one of the greatest risks for developing the major diseases of our time—diabetes, heart disease, cancer, infections, and arthritis—is allostatic load and abnormal stress hormone levels.

However critical to health proper food choices and dietary supplements are, they need to be supported by good self-care in other areas to maintain adaptation and well-being. After all, it is estimated that up to 75% of medical visits have a stress related component. Relaxation and adequate rest, meditation techniques, exercise and outdoor time, intimacy and laughter, time with friends and family, a rich spiritual life, healthy expression of emotions and needs, and health-fulfilling attitudes and behaviors are all part of adaptation and longevity. A detailed discussion of all these areas is beyond the scope of this book; however all of these areas are critical to maintain adaptation.

Exercise is such an important component of adaptation that it warrants a brief word. When I ask my patients what they do to decrease their stress, most reply that they work out at a gym or do other forms of aerobic exercise, the more intense the better. There certainly is benefit from aerobic exercise including improved insulin sensitivity and blood sugar levels, higher HDL cholesterol, lower total cholesterol, better weight management, and improved blood pressure. However, from the perspective of regulating cortisol, this is not always a great solution. In fact, the response to aerobic exercise or weight lifting is a temporary increase in cortisol, which is needed to reduce the inflammation triggered by the workout. This is why so many people who already might be marginal in their adrenal reserve do badly with this type of exercise.

If you feel that the result of an aerobic workout does relax you and doesn't trigger excess fatigue, then stick with it. However, for many people, walking at a brisk pace, low-intensity cycling, or swimming are better cortisol regulators. Better yet are yoga, *tai qi*, or *qi gong* techniques. These exercises directly improve cortisol function through breathing techniques, slow movement, *qi* generation, and a feeling of slowing down and grounding. Including one of these ancient arts with a meditation technique that can be done at home is a powerful approach to adaptation.

Beyond diet and exercise, changing the way you manage stress and how you think about stressful situations can have a dramatic adaptive impact. One example of the effect of attitudes on life experience is the quality of optimism. Optimists live longer, stay healthier, and are generally happier. Though optimism is considered a trait that one either possesses or doesn't, it is possible for anyone to adopt the qualities of optimists. Optimists take responsibility for their actions but not for what they can't control. Having a positive view of life events, optimists feel in control of their lives and expect success and happiness to be theirs. They feel they have the ability to fix what is wrong, deal more directly with stress, and eventually overcome difficult situations.

Another key attitude is feeling in control of one's life. Even more than other factors, maintaining a sense of control in a stressful situation can reduce allostatic load and help regain adaptation. The attitude that one can affect the course and destiny of one's life has been shown to improve healthy aging. A belief that difficult situations can be effectively managed reduces feelings of helplessness and hopelessness, leading to lower cortisol levels and improving resistance to many chronic diseases. Control means that you are not at the mercy of circumstances that you can't impact. At the very least, you can control your reaction to a situation.

Simple changes in attitudes like these can go a long way to adaptation and health. For some of my patients, adopting proper dietary practices was not possible because of underlying issues such as feeling out of control or being pessimistic. However, eating better brings about less depression and anxiety and empowers people to make the needed changes to maintain health. It is a classic chicken and egg phenomenon: poor control of cortisol leads to mental states that prevent some people from making the right choices to improve cortisol regulation, leading to continued allostatic load.

I have presented a very simple way of breaking out of this dilemma. If the first step can be taken by doing the initial elimination detoxification diet, then in the majority of people there will be an immediate reduction in allostatic load and better cortisol management. This often leads to less depression and a greater chance to make the long-term changes of the Adaptation Diet and succeed in controlling cortisol, losing weight, and increasing longevity.

Through measurement of salivary cortisol in many of my patients, I have been able to track improvement in their allostatic load from the Adaptation Diet. However, I don't think the average person needs to do cortisol testing to know when they are better adapted. As soon as the aches and pains reduce, digestive symptoms disappear, energy improves, and the mood stabilizes, you can be assured that biochemical adaptation is occurring. And as an extra bonus, losing weight generally follows improved adaptation. Reducing stress and cortisol through the Adaptation Diet is a step in maintaining health and aging well. Combining this with other effective self-care approaches is the answer to adaptation and health.

Appendix Outline

The appendix is divided into six sections to make it easier to apply the suggestions of the Adaptation Diet. Recipes are included for both the maintenance Adaptation Diet and specific requirements including yeast-free, wheat-free, and rotation diets.

Section 1: Glycemic Index

The glycemic index is a ranking of foods based on their effect on raising blood glucose levels. The index compares the level of blood sugar after eating a portion of food with the glucose levels after either straight glucose ingestion or a slice of white bread. The impact a food will have on blood sugar levels depends on other factors as well including the size of a standard portion, fiber content, and dietary fat levels. The glycemic index is meant to be a guide to food selection to be used in conjunction with other good dietary practices.

Section 2: Phases One and Two of the Adaptation Diet

A graph is included to help organize symptoms that might occur as you change your diet. Symptoms can occur from withdrawal from allergic foods. It is also useful to use this graph to track symptoms when foods are reintroduced during the challenge period of Phase Two.

Also included in this section are sample recipes of allowed foods during Phases One and Two of the Adaptation Diet. These recipes are from patient guides by Metagenics˙. Feel free to expand on these recipes as long as you adhere to the foods on the list on pages 23 and 24.

Section 3: Recipes for Phase Three, Maintenance Phase of the Adaptation Diet

Recipes included here are from a variety of sources. Nancy Brown, a skillful nutritionist, has worked with me for many years and kindly offered some menus ideas and recipes. Some of these recipes are from patient handouts designed by Metagenics'. In addition I have added selected recipes from Mediterranean diets that are widely available online and in multiple books. I have included a large variety of vegetarian recipes that should be used frequently in the Adaptation Diet.

Section 4: Rotation Diet

For those people who have identified multiple food allergies during the challenge phase, a rotation diet is essential to reduce allostatic load. I have included a sample four-day rotation program, menus, and shopping lists, kindly provided by Carol Buuck, as well as food-family charts. It is beyond the scope of this book to give all the needed information to be successful at rotating, but the American Academy of Environmental Medicine (see resources) has ample resources to help with this aspect of the diet. Rotation diets strongly regulate cortisol if done correctly.

Section 5: Wheat-free (Weigh Less)

If there is a concern about wheat allergy or gluten intolerance, I have included wheat and gluten-free recipes and a four-day rotation plan. All these recipes are from Nancy Brown, nutrition consultant. If there is a concern about celiac disease, consult your physician before making any dietary changes.

Section 6: Yeast-free

Many of my patients with food allergies and digestive problems do better on a yeast and wheat-free diet. If you tested positive to yeast in the food challenge or are curious whether you have *candida* overgrowth, a yeast-free diet will often enhance well-being in a few weeks. Included is the anti-yeast diet I use in my practice and suggestions on yeast-free foods.

Appendix Section 1

Glycemic Index

Slow Acting Low Glycemic	Moderately Acting Mdoerate Glycemic	Fast Acting High Glycemic
Breads: Rye kernel bread Barley kernel bread Whole-wheat kernel bread Multigrain bread	50% oat bran bread Whole-grain pumpernickel Cracked-wheat kernel bread Whole wheat	Rye-flour bread Bagels Pita bread White bread
Breakfast Cereals: All-Bran Rice bran	Toasted Muesli Oat bran Oatmeal (slow cooked)	Cheerios Bran Chex Instant Oatmeal Grapenuts Life Puffed Wheat Shredded Wheat Corn Flakes Cream of Wheat Nutri-Grain Chex
Cereal Grains: Barley Whole kernel wheat Whole kernel rye Long-grain parboiled rice	Cracked barley Bulgur Corn Brown rice	Rolled barley Buckwheat Cornmeal White rice Millet
Dairy: Unsweetened low-fat yogurt	Low-fat fruit yogurt	Frozen yogurt

Fruit:		
Apple	Apple juice (unsweetened)	Banana
Cherries	Grapes	Mango
Grapefruit	Orange	Orange juice
Peach	Dried apricots	Canned peaches in syrup
Pear	Canned pear in juice	Kiwi
Plum		Raisins
		Watermelon
		Pineapple
		Papaya
Legumes:		
Chickpeas	Canned chickpeas	Canned baked beans
Lentils	Black-eyed peas	Broad beans
Green beans	Pinto beans	Canned green beans
Red beans	Navy beans	Navy beans (pressure cooked 25 minutes)
Baby lima beans	Romano beans	
Kidney beans		
Soy Beans		
Split peas		
Pasta:		
Fettuccini, egg enriched	Capellini	Rice pasta, brown
Spaghetti, protein enriched	Spaghetti	Spaghetti (boiled 20 minutes)
Spaghetti, whole wheat	Macaroni (boiled 5 minutes)	Macaroni & Cheese (boxed)
Root Vegetables:		
	Yam	Beetroot
	Sweet potato	Carrots
		Parsnips
		Russet potato
		Instant potato
		New potato
		Sweet potato
		French fries
Vegetables:		
Dried peas	Green peas	Pumpkin
Dark leafy greens		Sweet corn
Soups:		
Tomato	Canned lentil	Black bean, canned
		Green pea, canned

Snack Foods: Peanuts Almonds Walnuts		Jelly beans Life Savers Mars Bars Muesli bars Popcorn Corn chips Potato chips Crackers Cookies
Sugars: Fructose	Lactose	Maltose Glucose Honey Sucrose

Appendix Section 2

Phase One and Two-Diet

This is a sample graph that can be used to track symptoms from withdrawal of allergic foods from the diet. It can also be used when these foods are reintroduced during the challenge period of Phase Two.

Symptom Chart

Instructions: Please grade the severity of your symptoms each day from 0 (none) to 10 (very severe).

Weight before starting: morning_____evening_____

Weight Day 10:   morning_____evening_____

Symptoms	Before	Day 1	Day 2	Day 3	Day 4	Day 5	Day 6	Day 7	Day 8	Day 9	Day 10
Headache											
Nausea											
Vomiting											
Abdominal pain											
Diarrhea											
Depression											
Irritability											
Insomnia											
Lethargy											
Backache											
Aching limbs											
Restless legs											
Morning resting pulse											

Sample Recipes for Phase One and Phase Two
(See page 27 for a list of allowed foods)

Beans and Greens Soup (4–5 servings)
2 T. olive oil
1 large onion, chopped
2 medium cloves garlic crushed
1 bay leaf
1–2 stalks celery, diced
1–2 medium carrots diced
1 t. salt
Black pepper to taste
5 cups water or vegetable broth
2 cups cooked white beans
½ lb. fresh chopped mixed greens: kale, collards, spinach, & escarole
Freshly grated nutmeg

In a saucepan, add oil and sauté the onions and garlic over low heat. When onions are soft, add celery, carrot, salt, and pepper. Stir and sauté another 5 minutes. Add broth or water and bay leaf. Cover and simmer about 20 minutes. Add cooked beans and greens. Cover and continue to simmer, over very low heat, another 15–20 minutes. Garnish as desired with grated nutmeg.

Kasha (serves 2)
1 t. olive oil
¼ cup chopped onion
1 celery stick, diced
½ cup uncooked kasha (buckwheat groats)
1 cup water
Salt and pepper to taste

Sauté onion and celery in oil. Add buckwheat and water and bring to boil. Reduce heat and simmer 20 minutes. Season with salt and pepper as desired.

Vegetable Dal Curry (serves 2)
1 t. olive oil
¼ cup chopped onion
1 t. turmeric powder

¼ t. coriander powder
Dash cumin
1 sliced carrot
1 cup cauliflower pieces
⅓ cup red lentils
1 cup water

Heat 1 t. olive oil and add ¼ cup onion, 1 t. turmeric powder, ¼ t. coriander powder, and a dash of cumin. Sauté. Add 1 sliced carrot and 1 cup of cauliflower pieces; stir to coat. Add ⅓ cup red lentils and 1 cup of water. Bring to a boil, reduce heat, and simmer about 40 minutes. Salt to taste.

Ratatouille (serves 6)
½ cup olive oil
2 large onions, sliced
3 garlic cloves, minced
1 medium eggplant cut into 1-inch cubes
2 green peppers, chopped
3 zucchini, cut into ½-inch slices
1 28-oz. can whole tomatoes, drained
1 t. salt
¼ t. pepper
1 t. oregano
½ t. thyme

In a 6-quart pot, sauté onion and garlic in oil for 3 minutes. Add eggplant and stir-fry for 5 minutes. Add peppers and cook 5 minutes. Add zucchini and cook for 5 more minutes. Add seasonings and tomatoes. Cover and simmer for 30 minutes.

Rice/Oat Pancakes (4–5 servings)
1 ½ cups rice milk
1 ½ T. lemon juice
1 ½ cups rice flour
½ cup oat flour
½ t. salt
2 t. baking powder
½ t. baking soda
1 T. apple butter
1 T. cold-pressed safflower oil
Egg substitute to equal 2 eggs

Mix rice milk and lemon juice together and allow to sit for 5 minutes until curds form. Mix dry ingredients together and set aside. In large mixing bowl, beat apple butter, oil, egg, and milk mixture. Add dry mixture and stir gently. Be careful not to overmix. Makes approximately 14 (4-inch) pancakes.

Cauliflower Salad (serves 10–12)
1 small head of cauliflower
3–4 cloves garlic, minced
½ cup chopped pecans
1 T. olive oil (for sautéing)
2 T. olive oil (for dressing)
2 T. flaxseed oil
2 T. vinegar
2 T. each freshly snipped parsley and chives
Salt and pepper to taste

Lightly steam cauliflower florets. Meanwhile, sauté garlic and pecans in 1 T. olive oil over very low heat until slightly brown. Mix with remaining oils, vinegar, and seasonings. In a large bowl, mix vegetables together and toss with garlic-pecan mixture. Add salt and pepper to taste. Flavor is enhanced the longer this salad sits.

Lentil Salad (serves 4)
⅔ cup uncooked lentils, well rinsed
2 cups water
1 bay leaf
1 T. chopped fresh basil or 1 t. dried basil
¼ cup finely diced red or green onions
1 whole carrot, grated
¼ cup finely chopped black olives
¼ cup raisins or currants
3 T. olive oil
1 T. balsamic vinegar

Simmer lentils and bay leaf in water for about 25 minutes or until tender. Drain and discard bay leaf. In a large bowl, gently toss lentils with basil, onions, grated carrot, chopped olives, and raisins or currants. Mix in Basic Salad and Veggie Dressing (follows) to taste. Gently toss and serve slightly chilled or at room temperature.

Semi-Greek Salad (serves 4)

3 cups mixed green
½ cup each shredded carrot, cabbage, green onions
1 cup cooked garbanzo beans
Few sliced black olives
Few red onion ringlets

Toss together all ingredients. Mix Basic Salad and Veggie Dressing (follows), making sure to add dry mustard, and toss with greens and veggies.

Basic Salad and Veggie Dressing (serves 6)

Mix well in a shaker jar (store any leftovers in refrigerator – dressing will solidify in the fridge):
¼ cup each flaxseed and olive oils
3-4 T. vinegar (apple cider, tarragon, rice, red wine, balsamic, ume plum)
1 T. water
Garlic, whole cloves or minced
Oregano, basil or other herbs of choice to taste
1 t. dry mustard (optional) whisked into liquid

Oat Bran Muffins (serves 8)

¾ cup almond milk
1 T. lemon juice
½ cup oat bran
1 ¾ cups whole oats
1 t. baking powder
½ t. baking soda
¼ t. salt
¼ cup chopped walnuts or almonds
¾ cup unsweetened applesauce
½ cup dates or dried apples

Preheat oven to 400 degrees. Spray muffin cups with oil and set aside. Combine almond milk and lemon juice in a cup and allow to set about 10 minutes or until curdles form. Combine dry ingredients in a large bowl. Add almond milk/lemon juice combination and applesauce, mixing gently with a spoon until completely moistened. Stir in dried fruit but do not overmix. Spoon into prepared muffin tin, filling about ¾ full. Bake 20–25 minutes until lightly browned. Allow to cool for 10 minutes before removing from pan.

Split Pea Soup (serves 6)

3 cups dry split peas
2 quarts water
1 bay leaf
2 onions, finely chopped
4 cloves garlic, minced
3 stalks celery, diced
2 medium carrots, sliced
Salt and black pepper to taste
3 T. apple cider or rice vinegar

Place ingredients in Dutch oven. Bring to boil and lower heat to simmer partially covered for about 60 minutes, stirring occasionally. Add more water as needed. Add pepper, salt, and vinegar to taste.

Quinoa Vegetable Soup (serves 4–6)

4 cups water
¼ cup quinoa (well rinsed)
½ cup carrots, diced
¼ cup celery, diced
2 T. onion, chopped
¼ cup green pepper, diced
2 cloves garlic, chopped
1 t. olive oil
½ cup tomatoes, chopped
½ cup cabbage, chopped
1 t. salt

Sauté quinoa, carrots, celery, onions, green pepper, and garlic in oil until golden brown. Add water, tomatoes, and cabbage and bring to a boil. Simmer 20 to 30 minutes or until tender. Season to taste and garnish with parsley.

For variations, try adding some of your other favorite vegetables, chopped and sautéed.

Millet Pate (serves 4)

½ cup cooked millet
½ cup silken extra-firm tofu
¼ cup grated carrot
1 T. tahini
1 ½ T. light yellow miso

3 T. nutritional yeast
⅛ t. each celery seed and savory

Place all ingredients in a bowl and mix well. Serve as a spread on rice cakes.

Stir-Fry Vegetables and Chicken (serves 2)

1 t. sesame oil
2 t. grated fresh ginger
Any combination of the following vegetables:

> 2 carrots, diced
> 1 stalk celery, diced
> 1 cup bok choy, chopped
> ½ cup diced onion
> ½ cup chopped broccoli and/or cauliflower
> ½ cup snow peas
> ¼ cup mung bean sprouts

3 oz. boneless organic chicken, cut into strips or cubes
Freshly chopped basil to taste
1 t. flaxseed oil

Heat sesame oil and ginger in a wok and stir-fry your choice of vegetables for about 5 minutes. Add chicken pieces and continue to stir-fry until cooked through. Optional: Just before removing from heat, add freshly chopped basil. Add 1 t. flaxseed oil upon completion of cooking. Serve with Pecan Rice.

Pecan Rice (serves 4)

1 cup wild and brown rice mix
2 ½ cups water
2 T. chopped pecans
1 t. walnut or olive oil

Bring water to a boil and add rice, stirring to mix well. Cover and simmer rice for about 45 minutes or until all liquid has been absorbed. Do not stir while cooking. While rice is cooking, sauté pecans in oil over low heat until lightly browned. Toss pecan mixture with cooked rice and serve immediately.

Sassy Beans (serves 1)
1 t. olive oil
1 T. chopped scallions
1 clove garlic, minced
½ cup chopped onion
½ cup vegetarian refried beans
¼ cup cilantro, chopped
Chopped black olives
¼ of an avocado

Sauté scallions, garlic, and onion in olive oil. Add refried beans. Remove from heat and garnish with optional cilantro, black olives, and avocado. Serve with Pecan Rice.

Appendix Section 3

Recipes for Maintenance Phase Three of The Adaptation Diet

V = vegetarian

Vegan Roasted Red Pepper Hummus (*V) (serves 6–8)
1 15-oz. can chickpeas (garbanzo beans), drained
1 roasted red pepper (see notes below)
3 T. lemon juice
½ T. sesame tahini
1 clove garlic, minced
½ t. ground cumin
½ t. red chili powder or cayenne pepper

Puree chickpeas, roasted red pepper, lemon juice, sesame tahini, garlic, cumin, and red chili powder together in a blender or food processor. It should be thick and smooth but grainy. Add kosher salt to taste. If serving as dip, drizzle with extra virgin olive oil before serving.

Recipe Notes: For the roasted red pepper, you can either buy them canned (or in a jar), or you can simply grill or broil them until black on each side. Once they cool, the blackened outside simply rubs off.

Summer Chicken Salad with Garden Herbs (serves 6–8)
1 3 ½ lb. whole chicken
¼ cup chopped fresh chives
3 T. white or red wine vinegar
2 T. capers
2 T. thyme
1 t. oregano

4 t. extra virgin olive oil
½ t. salt, preferably sea salt
½ t. fresh ground pepper
2 cloves garlic, minced

Place chicken in a stockpot; cover with water and bring to a boil. Reduce heat and simmer 50 minutes or until tender. Drain, reserving broth for another use. Cool chicken completely. Remove skin from chicken and discard. Remove chicken from bones and discard bones and fat. Chop chicken into bite-sized pieces.

Combine chives and remaining ingredients in a large bowl. Add chicken; toss well to coat.

Recipe Notes: To save 50 minutes of cooking time, just stop by the grocery store and pick up a chicken that's already roasted. This is a huge time saver and delicious too.

Mediterranean Chicken and Rice Bake (serves 6)
1 ¾ cups chicken broth
¼ cup chopped fresh parsley
¼ cup sliced pitted ripe olives
1 T. lemon juice
¼ t. ground black pepper
1 can (about 14 ½ oz.) stewed tomatoes
1 ¼ cups uncooked regular long-grain brown rice
6 skinless, boneless chicken breasts
½ t. garlic powder
Paprika

Mix broth, parsley, olives, lemon juice, black pepper, tomatoes, and rice in 3-qt. shallow baking dish. Cover. Bake at 375 degrees for 20 min.

Top with chicken. Sprinkle with garlic powder and paprika. Bake an additional 30 minutes or until chicken and rice are done.

Grilled Salmon with Mustard and Herbs (serves 3–4)
2 lemons, thinly sliced, plus 1 lemon cut into wedges for garnish
20-30 springs mixed fresh herbs
2 T. chopped mixed herbs
1 clove garlic

¼ t. salt
1 T. Dijon mustard
1 lb. center-cut salmon, skinned (see Tip)

Preheat grill to medium-high.

Lay two 9-inch pieces of heavy-duty foil on top of each other and place on a rimless baking sheet. Arrange lemon slices in two layers in the center of the foil. Spread herb sprigs over the lemons. With the side of a chef's knife, mash garlic with salt to form a paste. Transfer to a small dish and stir in mustard and the remaining 2 T. chopped herbs. Spread the mixture over both sides of the salmon. Place the salmon on the herb sprigs.

Slide the foil and salmon off the baking sheet onto the grill without disturbing the salmon-lemon stack. Cover the grill; cook until the salmon is opaque in the center, 18 to 24 minutes. Wearing oven mitts, carefully transfer foil and salmon back onto the baking sheet. Cut the salmon into 4 portions and serve with lemon wedges (discard herb sprigs and lemon slices).

Tip: To skin a salmon fillet, place salmon fillet on a clean cutting board, skin-side down. Starting at the tail end, slip the blade of a long knife between the fish flesh and the skin, holding down firmly with your other hand. Gently push the blade along at a 30° angle, separating the fillet from the skin without cutting through either.

Asian Gazpacho (*V) (serves 6)
6 tomatoes, seeded and finely chopped, or 1 28-oz. can chopped tomatoes
2 cups vegetable broth
1 t. dry sherry
2 T. fresh cilantro, chopped
1 T. light soy sauce
4 scallions, white part only
4 thin slivers of fresh ginger
¼–½ t. Chinese chili sauce, to taste
2 limes

Place the tomatoes, over low heat, in a 2 or 3-quart saucepan. Add in the vegetable broth, sherry, cilantro, soy sauce, scallions, and ginger. Bring the mixture to a simmer and cook for 20 minutes. Remove from the heat and allow to cool for a few minutes. Puree in a food processor or blender. Chill.

Just before serving, stir in chili sauce. Grate the peel of one lime and add to the soup. Squeeze the juice from both of the limes into the soup.

Creamy Cold Tomato Soup (*V) (serves 5)
1 cucumber, chopped
1 scallion, chopped
1 clove garlic
4 cups tomato juice
1 green pepper, chopped
½ t. dill weed
Sliced mushrooms or tomato chunks for garnish
1 cup plain yogurt

Combine all ingredients (except yogurt) in small amounts in blender and blend until smooth. Use salt sparingly, if needed, and add pepper. Whisk in yogurt. Chill several hours before serving and garnish as desired with mushrooms or tomatoes.

Hummus Wrap (serves 1)
2 small or 1 large low-carb tortilla(s)
¼ cup hummus
8–10 cherry tomatoes
¼ avocado, slivered

Spread 2 T. hummus on each tortilla. Top with 4–5 cherry tomatoes on each and garnish with slivers of avocado.

Cold Salmon with Raita (serves 8)
2 pounds salmon fillets (about 1 ½ inches thick)
1–2 T. olive oil

Preheat oven to 275 degrees. Place salmon skin-side down in ovenproof pan. Brush with olive oil. Roast uncovered until salmon flakes with a fork, about 25–30 minutes. Do not allow it to overcook. Serve at room temperature. Make a day ahead and refrigerate, but bring to room temperature before serving. Serve topped with Raita (recipe follows).

Raita (serves 8)
⅛ t. salt
1 cucumber, chopped into small dice
1 tomato, chopped into small dice

1 medium carrot, grated
¼ cup chopped onion
1 cup plain, low-fat yogurt
2–3 T. chopped fresh cilantro or mint or 1 t. ground cumin (optional)

In a mixing bowl, mix cucumbers, carrots, and tomatoes with salt and allow to sit for 15–30 minutes. Drain well. Combine with yogurt and optional ingredient, if desired. Chill for 20 minutes. Serve with salmon.

Crustless Vegetable Quiche (serves 8)
5 eggs
½ cup non-fat or 1% low-fat milk
12 oz. (¾ cup) non-fat or low-fat cottage cheese
½ cup grated part-skim mozzarella cheese
10 oz. frozen chopped broccoli, thawed
10 oz. frozen chopped spinach, thawed
1 T. olive oil
½ t. salt
¼ t. fresh ground pepper

Beat eggs in a medium-sized bowl. Add milk and beat some more. Add remaining ingredients and stir vigorously to blend. Pour into a deep, lightly oiled casserole, and place it in a 9 x 13-inch pan filled partway with hot water. Bake in a 375 degree oven for about 35–45 minutes, or until a knife, inserted into center of the quiche, comes out clean.

Fish Creole (serves 4)
1 T. olive oil
1 onion, chopped
½ cup thin-sliced celery
¼ cup green pepper, chopped
1 garlic clove, minced
2 T. fresh parsley or 2 t. dried
1 bay leaf
¼ t. rosemary, chopped
1 28-oz. can tomatoes with liquid
1 pound fish fillets
2 cups cooked brown rice

Heat oil in a large saucepan and lightly sauté the onion, celery, pepper, and garlic until soft. Add parsley, bay leaf, rosemary, and tomatoes. Simmer, uncovered, about 20 minutes. Add fish fillets in small pieces and simmer until cooked through, about 5–10 minutes more. Remove bay leaf. Serve over brown rice.

Grilled Leg of Lamb (serves 4 per pound)
1 leg of lamb (boned and butterflied by butcher)
2 cups red wine
2 t. poultry seasoning
1 t. salt
3 cloves garlic, cut in slivers

Mix ingredients and marinate for 12–24 hours in refrigerator.

Grill over hot coals approximately 20 minutes on each side. Baste occasionally while grilling. This is a delicious replacement for steak!

Lentil-Barley Stew (*V) (serves 8)
2 T. olive oil
4 medium carrots, diced
2 medium leeks (with 3 inches of green left on), diced
2 celery stalks, diced
2 medium zucchini, diced
1 large onion, diced
2 garlic cloves, minced
1 t. dried thyme
1 cup dried lentils, rinsed
½ cup barley
6–8 cups chicken or vegetable broth
2 cups diced tomatoes
1 cup chopped fresh basil leaves
½ cup chopped parsley
Salt and pepper to taste

Heat olive oil in a large heavy pot and add carrots, leeks, celery, zucchini, onion, and garlic. Cook over low heat, stirring occasionally, for about 10 minutes until vegetables have softened. Add lentils, barley, thyme, and 6 cups broth. Bring to a boil and reduce heat to a simmer. Cook uncovered about 30 minutes, stirring often. Add remaining 2 cups of broth as needed if dry. Add tomatoes and basil and salt and pepper to taste; cook 10 more minutes. Stir in parsley and serve.

Mango Salmon (serves 6)
2 t. tamari or regular soy sauce
1 T. fresh ginger, minced
1 cinnamon stick (3 inches)
1 t. rice or cider vinegar
1 10-oz. bottle mango nectar
6 salmon fillets, 5 oz. each and 1 inch thick
1 t. olive oil

In a small saucepan, stir together all ingredients, except for salmon. Bring to boil, reduce heat, and simmer uncovered for 20–25 minutes or until reduced to about ¾ cup. Pour mixture through a strainer and discard the solids. Return to saucepan and keep warm.

Brush olive oil on broiler pan, place salmon on pan, and broil 5 inches away from heat for 5 minutes. Brush salmon with mango mixture and broil 3 more minutes or until fish flakes with a fork. Serve immediately and allow individuals to garnish salmon with remaining mixture as desired.

Roasted Salmon or Red Snapper with Salsa (serves 8)
4 salmon or red snapper fillets, 8 oz. each
4 t. olive oil
1 T. fresh lime juice
1 T. fresh cilantro, chopped
Salt and pepper to taste

Preheat oven to 400 degrees. Brush 1 t. olive oil on a baking sheet and place fish skin-side down. Combine remaining olive oil, lime juice, and cilantro; brush on each fillet. Sprinkle with salt and pepper to taste. Allow to sit for 15 minutes, then bake for 20 minutes or until just cooked. Garnish with Salsa (recipe follows) and serve immediately.

Salsa (serves 1)
Combine in a bowl:
2 large tomatoes, diced
2 scallions, chopped
1 T. cilantro, chopped
1 clove garlic, chopped
1 T. olive oil
2 t. fresh lime juice

Spaghetti Squash Topped with Ratatouille (serves 6)
One medium spaghetti squash, halved with seeds removed.

Place squash cut-side up in an ovenproof dish with ½ inch water and cover with foil. Bake at 375 degrees for about 40 minutes or until easily pierced with a fork. Do not overbake. When squash is cool enough to handle, scrape with a fork to release spaghettilike strands. Top with Ratatouille (recipe follows).

Ratatouille (*V) (serves 6)
¼ cup olive oil
2 large onions, sliced
3 garlic cloves, minced
1 medium eggplant, cut into 1-inch cubes
2 green peppers, chopped
3 zucchini, cut into ½-inch slices
1 28-oz. can tomatoes, drained (fresh, ripe tomatoes may be substituted when available)
1 t. salt
¼ t. pepper
1 t. oregano
½ t. thyme

In a 6-quart pot, sauté onion and garlic in 1 T. oil for 3 minutes. Add 1 T. oil and eggplant and stir-fry for 5 minutes. Add another T. oil and the peppers and cook 5 minutes. Add the last T. oil and the zucchini; cook for 5 more minutes. Then add seasonings and tomatoes; cover and simmer for 30 minutes. Use to top spaghetti squash or as a vegetable side dish.

Stir-Fried Tofu with Ginger Broccoli (*V) (serves 4)
1 pound extra-firm tofu
2 T. tamari (low-sodium soy sauce)
3 T. olive oil
2 t. peeled and minced fresh ginger
2 garlic cloves minced
2 cups broccoli florets
2 cups sliced mushrooms
1 red bell pepper cut into thin strips
1 T. arrowroot or cornstarch
1 T. dry sherry
½ t. cayenne or ¼ t. hot-pepper flakes
1 t. sesame oil

Slice tofu into cubes. Toss with tamari soy sauce and set aside for 5–10 minutes. In a wok or large nonstick skillet, heat 1 T. oil over high heat. When oil is hot, lower heat to medium-high and add scallions, ginger, and garlic; stir-fry for 30 seconds. Drain tofu, reserving tamari, and add tofu, stir-frying for 2 more minutes. Remove from pan and set aside.

Using a fork or small whisk, mix reserved tamari with arrowroot or cornstarch, sherry, and cayenne in a small bowl. Set aside.

Heat another 1 T. oil in wok over high heat. Add broccoli, mushrooms, and bell pepper, and stir-fry for 2 minutes. Add ¼ cup water and bring to boil. Cover wok and reduce heat to medium, steaming vegetables about 5 minutes until slightly tender. Return tofu to wok.

Stir reserved tamari mixture into wok, and cook over medium heat until thickened and thoroughly heated; do not overcook vegetables. Add sesame oil, salt, and pepper to taste, and adjust seasonings if you desire a spicier dish. Serve immediately or make ahead and refrigerate until ready to serve. Reheat carefully; flavors are enhanced when the dish sits overnight.

Tofu/Vegetable Stir-Fry (*V) (serves 4)

1 14-oz. package firm tofu, drained and cubed
1 T. fresh ginger, grated or chopped
2 cups any combination of chopped vegetables, such as bok choy, celery, bean sprouts, Napa cabbage, or blanched broccoli or cauliflower
1 T. sesame oil
1 clove garlic, chopped
1 cup sliced fresh mushrooms
1 red bell pepper, cut into strips
2–4 T. tamari (soy sauce)
2 cups cooked brown rice

Heat oil in wok over high heat; add garlic and ginger and stir constantly until lightly browned. Add vegetables and cook for 3 or 4 minutes, depending on crispness desired. Add tamari and cubed tofu; cook an additional minute; remove from heat. Serve over brown rice.

Turkey-Bulgur Skillet (*V) (serves 4)

1 lb. ground turkey or ¾ lb. cubed tofu
1 medium onion, chopped
1 clove garlic, minced

1 cup uncooked bulgur wheat
1 16-oz. canned tomatoes, including juice
1 cup water
¼ t. marjoram
½ t. thyme
2 bay leaves
1 ½ cups frozen peas, defrosted
Salt and pepper to taste

In a large, heavy skillet over medium heat, sauté turkey, onion, and garlic until onion is softened. Drain off excess fat. Add bulgur and cook for one minute more. Stir in tomatoes, water, and spices. Cover and simmer for 20 minutes, stirring occasionally to break up tomatoes. Add peas, and salt and pepper to taste.

(**Vegetarian option**: Omit turkey and sauté the onion and garlic in 2 t. olive oil. Add ¾ lb. of cubed tofu to the skillet along with the bulgur.)

Turkey Chili (*V) (serves 8)
2 lbs. ground turkey
2 16-oz. cans tomatoes, cut up (undrained)
2 15-oz. cans red kidney beans, drained
1 8-oz. can tomato sauce
1 medium onion, chopped
1 t. dried parsley flakes
¾ t. dried basil, crushed
¾ t. dried oregano, crushed
½ t. black pepper
½ t. ground cinnamon
1 clove garlic, minced
¼ cup dry red wine, optional
¼–½ t. ground red pepper
1–2 T. chili powder
1 bay leaf

In a 4-quart Dutch oven cook the turkey until it is no longer pink. Drain off fat. Stir in undrained tomatoes, drained kidney beans, tomato sauce, onion, wine (if desired), and spices. Simmer uncovered for 45 minutes, stirring occasionally.

Vegetarian option: Omit turkey and add 2 cups cauliflower pieces, 1 large chopped potato, 1 chopped green bell pepper, 2 chopped carrots, ½ lb. chopped mushrooms, and 3 cups fresh or frozen corn kernels to the ingredients listed above. Bring mixture to a boil. Simmer uncovered until vegetables are tender, about 30 minutes.

Mediterranean Fish Fillets (serves 2)
1 t. extra-virgin olive oil
1 small onion, thinly sliced
2 T. dry white wine
1 clove garlic, finely chopped
1 cup canned diced tomatoes
4 Kalamata olives, pitted and chopped
⅛ t. dried oregano
⅛ t. freshly grated orange zest
¼ t. salt, divided
¼ t. freshly ground pepper, divided
8 oz. thick-cut, firm-fleshed fish fillets, such as Pacific halibut or mahi-mahi

Preheat oven to 450 degrees. Heat oil in a medium nonstick skillet over medium-high heat. Add onion and cook, stirring often, until lightly browned, 2 to 4 minutes. Add wine and garlic and simmer for 30 seconds. Stir in tomatoes, olives, oregano, and orange zest. Season with ⅛ teaspoon salt and ⅛ teaspoon pepper.

Season fish with the remaining ⅛ teaspoon each salt and pepper. Arrange the fish in a single layer in a pie pan or baking dish. Spoon the tomato mixture over the fish. Bake, uncovered, until the fish is just cooked through, 10 to 20 minutes. Divide the fish into 2 portions and serve with sauce.

Mediterranean Lamb Salad (serves 6)
1 pound boneless leg of lamb steaks, 1–1 ½ inches thick
1 ½ t. kosher salt, divided
Freshly ground pepper to taste
2 medium cucumbers, peeled, halved, seeded, and diced
2 large tomatoes, diced
1 15-oz. can chickpeas, rinsed
½ cup minced red onion
¼ cup crumbled feta cheese
¼ cup sliced fresh mint leaves

¼ cup lemon juice
1 t. extra-virgin olive oil

Preheat grill to high. Sprinkle lamb with ½ t. salt and pepper. Grill the lamb for 2–4 minutes per side for medium, depending on the thickness of the steaks. Transfer to a cutting board and let rest for at least 5 minutes before thinly slicing across the grain.

Meanwhile, place cucumbers, tomatoes, chickpeas, onion, feta cheese, and mint in a large bowl. Add lemon juice, oil, the remaining 1 t. salt, and more pepper to taste; stir to combine. Serve topped with the sliced lamb.

Middle Eastern Chickpea and Rice Stew (serves 6)
1 T. extra-virgin olive oil
3 medium onions, halved and thinly sliced (about 3 cups)
2 t. ground cumin
2 t. ground coriander
1 cup orange juice
4 cups reduced-sodium chicken broth or vegetable broth
2 15-oz. cans chickpeas, rinsed
3 cups peeled and diced sweet potato (about 1 pound)
⅔ cup brown basmati rice
¼ t. salt
¼ t. freshly ground pepper
½ cup chopped fresh cilantro

Heat oil in a large saucepan over medium heat; add onions and cook, stirring often, until tender and well browned, 10–12 minutes. Add cumin and coriander and stir for about 15 seconds. Add orange juice and broth. Stir in chickpeas, sweet potato, rice, and salt. Bring to a boil; reduce heat to a gentle simmer and cover. Cook, stirring occasionally, until the rice is tender and the sweet potatoes are breaking down to thicken the liquid, about 45 minutes. Season with pepper. (The stew will be thick and will thicken further upon standing. Add more broth to thin, if desired, or when reheating.) Serve topped with cilantro.

Mustard-Crusted Salmon (serves 4)
1 ¼ lbs. center-cut salmon fillets, cut into 4 portions
¼ t. salt, or to taste
Freshly ground pepper to taste
¼ cup reduced-fat sour cream

2 T. stone-ground mustard
2 t. lemon juice
Lemon wedges

Preheat broiler. Line a broiler pan or baking sheet with foil, then coat it with cooking spray. Place salmon pieces, skin-side down, on the prepared pan. Season with salt and pepper. Combine sour cream, mustard, and lemon juice in a small bowl. Spread evenly over the salmon.

Broil the salmon 5 inches from the heat source until it is opaque in the center, 10–12 minutes. Serve with lemon wedges.

Roasted Cod with Warm Tomato-Olive-Caper Tapenade (serves 4)
1 pound cod fillet
3 t. extra-virgin olive oil, divided
¼ t. freshly ground pepper
1 T. minced shallot
1 cup halved cherry tomatoes
¼ cup chopped cured olives
1 T. capers, rinsed and chopped
1 ½ t. chopped fresh oregano
1 t. balsamic vinegar

Preheat oven to 450 degrees. Coat a baking sheet with cooking spray. Rub cod with 2 t. oil. Sprinkle with pepper. Place on the prepared baking sheet. Transfer to the oven and roast until the fish flakes easily with a fork, 15–20 minutes, depending on the thickness of the fillet.

Meanwhile, heat the remaining 1 t. oil in a small skillet over medium heat. Add shallot and cook, stirring, until it begins to soften, about 20 seconds. Add tomatoes and cook, stirring, until softened, about 1 ½ minutes. Add olives and capers; cook, stirring, for 30 seconds more. Stir in oregano and vinegar; remove from heat. Spoon the tapenade over the cod to serve.

Seafood Couscous Paella (serves 2)
2 t. extra-virgin olive oil
1 medium onion, chopped
1 clove garlic, minced
½ t. dried thyme
½ t. fennel seed
¼ t. salt

¼ t. freshly ground pepper
Pinch of crumbled saffron threads
1 cup no-salt-added diced tomatoes, with juice
¼ cup vegetable broth
4 oz. bay scallops, tough muscle removed
4 oz. small shrimp (41–50 per pound), peeled and deveined
½ cup whole-wheat couscous

Heat oil in a large saucepan over medium heat. Add onion; cook, stirring constantly, for 3 minutes. Add garlic, thyme, fennel seed, salt, pepper, and saffron; cook for 20 seconds.

Stir in tomatoes and broth. Bring to a simmer. Cover, reduce heat, and simmer for 2 minutes.

Increase heat to medium, stir in scallops, and cook, stirring occasionally, for 2 minutes. Add shrimp and cook, stirring occasionally, for 2 minutes more. Stir in couscous. Cover, remove from heat, and let stand for 5 minutes; fluff.

Spiced Turkey with Avocado-Grapefruit Relish (serves 2)
Avocado-Grapefruit Relish
1 large seedless grapefruit
½ small avocado, peeled, pitted, and diced
1 small shallot, minced
1 T. chopped fresh cilantro
1 t. red-wine vinegar
1 t. honey
Spiced Turkey
1 T. chili powder
½ t. Chinese five-spice powder
⅛ t. salt
2 turkey cutlets (8 oz.)
1 T. canola oil

To prepare relish: Remove the peel and white pith from grapefruit with a sharp knife and discard. Cut the grapefruit segments from the surrounding membrane, letting them drop into a small bowl. Squeeze out remaining juice into the bowl and discard membrane. Add avocado, shallot, cilantro, vinegar, and honey. Toss well to combine.

To prepare turkey: Combine chili powder, five-spice powder, and salt on a plate. Dredge turkey in the spice mixture.

Heat oil in a medium skillet over medium-high heat. Add the turkey and cook until no longer pink in the middle, about 2–3 minutes per side. Serve the turkey with the avocado-grapefruit relish.

Butternut Squash Pilaf (*V) (serves 8)

2 pounds butternut squash, peeled, halved, and seeded
3 T. extra-virgin olive oil
1 large red onion, finely chopped
1 clove garlic, minced
2 T. water
1 T. tomato paste
1 cup instant or parboiled brown rice
1 ¾ cups water or 1 14-oz. can vegetable broth
½ cup white wine
½ cup chopped fennel fronds
2 T. chopped fresh oregano
1 t. salt
Pinch of cinnamon
Freshly ground pepper to taste

Grate the squash through the large holes of a box grater.

Heat oil in a large cast-iron or nonstick skillet over medium-low heat. Add onion and garlic and cook, stirring, until soft and lightly colored, 10–12 minutes. Combine 2 T. water and tomato paste in a small bowl and stir it into the pan. Add rice and stir to coat. Add the squash, in batches if necessary, and stir until it has reduced in volume enough so that you can cover the pan.

Increase the heat to medium-high, pour in 1 ¾ cups water (or broth) and wine, cover, and bring to a boil. Reduce the heat to medium-low and cook, covered, stirring once or twice, until the rice has absorbed most of the liquid and the squash is tender, 25–30 minutes.

Add fennel fronds, oregano, salt, cinnamon, and pepper; gently stir to combine. Remove from the heat and let stand, covered, for 5 minutes. Serve hot or at room temperature.

Lima Bean Spread with Cumin and Herbs (*V) (serves 6–8)
1 10-oz. package frozen lima beans
4 cloves garlic, crushed and peeled
¼ t. crushed red pepper
2 T. extra-virgin olive oil
4 t. lemon juice
1 t. ground cumin
½ t. salt, or to taste
Freshly ground pepper to taste
1 T. chopped fresh mint
1 T. chopped fresh cilantro
1 T. chopped fresh dill

Bring a large saucepan of lightly salted water to a boil. Add lima beans, garlic, and crushed red pepper; cook until the beans are tender, about 10 minutes. Remove from heat and let cool in the liquid.

Drain the beans and garlic. Transfer to a food processor. Add oil, lemon juice, cumin, salt, and pepper; process until smooth. Scrape into a bowl; stir in mint, cilantro, and dill. Good as veggie dip or spread on crackers, etc.

Parsley Tabbouleh (*V) (serves 4)
1 cup water
½ cup bulgur
¼ cup lemon juice
2 T. extra-virgin olive oil
½ t. minced garlic
¼ t. salt
Freshly ground pepper to taste
2 cups finely chopped flat-leaf parsley (about 2 bunches)
¼ cup chopped fresh mint
2 tomatoes, diced
1 small cucumber, peeled, seeded, and diced
4 scallions, thinly sliced

Combine water and bulgur in a small saucepan. Bring to a full boil, remove from heat, cover, and let stand until the water is absorbed and the bulgur is tender, 25 minutes or according to package directions. If any water remains, drain bulgur in a fine-mesh sieve. Transfer to a large bowl and let cool for 15 minutes.

Combine lemon juice, oil, garlic, salt, and pepper in a small bowl. Add parsley, mint, tomatoes, cucumber, and scallions to the bulgur. Add the dressing and toss. Serve at room temperature or chill for at least 1 hour to serve cold.

Ratatouille à la Casablancaise (*V) (serves 8)

1 large eggplant (1 ¼–1 ½ lbs.), peeled and cut into ¼-inch cubes
1 ½ t. salt, divided
3 T. plus 1 t. extra-virgin olive oil, divided
1 medium yellow summer squash, peeled and cut into ¼-inch cubes
1 red bell pepper, diced
3 medium tomatoes, peeled, seeded, and diced, or 1 cup drained canned diced tomatoes
2 cloves garlic, minced
1 ¼ t. ground cinnamon
1 t. sugar
¼ t. freshly ground pepper

Place eggplant on a baking sheet and sprinkle with 1 t. salt; let stand for 30 minutes. Rinse and pat dry.

Heat 3 T. oil in a nonstick skillet over medium-high heat. Add the eggplant, squash, and bell pepper. Cook, stirring, until the vegetables are soft, 8–10 minutes. Transfer to a large bowl.

Add the remaining 1 t. oil to the pan. Add tomatoes, garlic, cinnamon, sugar, the remaining ½ t. salt, and pepper. Cook, stirring, until the tomatoes begin to break down, 3–5 minutes. Add to the bowl with the eggplant mixture, and stir to combine. Cool to room temperature before serving for the best flavor.

Red-Wine Risotto (*V) (serves 8)

4 ½ cups reduced-sodium beef broth
2 T. extra-virgin olive oil
1 medium onion, finely chopped
2 cloves garlic, minced
1 ½ cups arborio, carnaroli, or other Italian "risotto" rice
¼ t. salt
1 ¾ cups dry red wine, such as Barbera, Barbaresco, or Pinot Noir
2 t. tomato paste
1 cup finely shredded Parmigiano-Reggiano cheese, divided
Freshly ground pepper to taste

Place broth in a medium saucepan; bring to a simmer over medium-high heat. Reduce the heat so the broth remains steaming but is not simmering.

Heat oil in a Dutch oven over medium-low heat. Add onion and cook, stirring occasionally, for 5 minutes. Add garlic and cook, stirring, until the onion is very soft and translucent, about 2 minutes. Add rice and salt and stir to coat.

Stir ½ cup of the hot broth and a generous splash of wine into the rice; reduce heat to a gentle simmer and cook, stirring constantly, until the liquid has been absorbed. Add more broth, ½ cup at a time along with some wine, stirring after each addition until most of the liquid has been absorbed. After about 10 minutes, stir in tomato paste. Continue to cook, adding broth and wine and stirring after each addition until most of the liquid is absorbed; the risotto is done when you've used all the broth and wine and the rice is creamy and just tender, 20–30 minutes more.

Remove the risotto from the heat; stir in ¾ cup cheese and pepper. Serve sprinkled with the remaining ¼ cup cheese.

Roasted Root Vegetables with Chermoula (*V) (serves 6)
¼ cup extra-virgin olive oil
3 cloves garlic, minced
2 t. paprika, preferably sweet Hungarian
2 t. ground cumin
1 t. salt
1 medium baking potato, peeled and cut into 1-inch chunks
1 medium sweet potato, peeled and cut into 1-inch chunks
1 medium turnip, peeled and cut into 1-inch chunks
1 medium rutabaga, peeled and cut into 1-inch chunks
2 medium carrots, cut into ½-inch slices
8 oz. peeled and seeded butternut squash, cut into 1-inch chunks

Preheat oven to 425 degrees. Place oil, garlic, paprika, cumin, and salt in a food processor or blender and pulse or blend until smooth.

Place potato, sweet potato, turnip, rutabaga, carrots, and squash in a roasting pan large enough to accommodate the pieces in a single layer. Toss with the spiced oil mixture until well combined.

Roast the vegetables, stirring once or twice, until tender, 45–50 minutes.

Roasted Eggplant and Feta Dip (*V) (serves 12)
1 medium eggplant (about 1 pound)
2 T. lemon juice
¼ cup extra-virgin olive oil
½ cup crumbled feta cheese, preferably Greek
½ cup finely chopped red onion
1 small red bell pepper, finely chopped
1 small chili pepper, such as jalapeño, seeded and minced (optional)
2 T. chopped fresh basil
1 T. finely chopped flat-leaf parsley
¼ t. cayenne pepper, or to taste
¼ t. salt
Pinch of sugar (optional)

Position oven rack about 6 inches from the heat source; preheat broiler.

Line a baking pan with foil. Place eggplant in the pan and poke a few holes all over it to vent steam. Broil the eggplant, turning with tongs every 5 minutes, until the skin is charred and a knife inserted into the dense flesh near the stem goes in easily, 14–18 minutes. Transfer to a cutting board until cool enough to handle.

Put lemon juice in a medium bowl. Cut the eggplant in half lengthwise and scrape the flesh into the bowl, tossing with the lemon juice to help prevent discoloring. Add oil and stir with a fork until the oil is absorbed. (It should be a little chunky.) Stir in feta, onion, bell pepper, chili pepper (if using), basil, parsley, cayenne, and salt. Taste and add sugar if needed.

Sautéed Spinach with Pine Nuts and Golden Raisins (*V) (serves 2)
2 t. extra-virgin olive oil
2 T. golden raisins
1 T. pine nuts
2 cloves garlic, minced
1 10-oz. bag fresh spinach, tough stems removed
2 t. balsamic vinegar
⅛ t. salt
1 T. shaved Parmesan cheese
Freshly ground pepper to taste

Heat oil in a large nonstick skillet or Dutch oven over medium-high heat. Add raisins, pine nuts, and garlic; cook, stirring, until fragrant, about 30 seconds. Add spinach and cook, stirring, until just wilted, about 2 minutes. Remove from heat; stir in vinegar and salt. Serve immediately, sprinkle with Parmesan and pepper.

Adzuki Bean Soup (*V) (serves 4–6)

3 cups Adzuki beans
1 small onion diced
3 small stalks celery diced
1 ear corn (optional)
2 T. garlic, chopped
1 T. Spike
1 T. Chinese five-spice powder
Sea salt (unrefined) to taste
1 ½ T. molasses
¼ cup tomato paste
⅓ cup cilantro, chopped
Arrowroot as needed

Soak beans overnight and discard water. Add fresh water and cook beans until tender. In a separate pan cook onions and celery over medium heat until tender. Then add corn, garlic, Spike, Chinese five-spice powder, molasses, and tomato paste and simmer for 10 minutes. Add this mixture to the cooked beans. (Hint: Remove and reserve some of the beans' water to adjust consistency later.) Bring soup to a simmer and thicken with an arrowroot slurry. Adjust flavor with salt to taste. Add cilantro at the very end.

Crusty Herbed Cauliflower (*V) (serves 4-6)

1 medium cauliflower head (about 2 pounds)
2 eggs
½ t. sea salt
1 T. Spike
1 cup bread crumbs (dry and whole grain)
½ cup fresh chopped basil
¼ cup parsley leaves, chopped
3 T. wheat flour
1 T. butter, melted

Preheat oven to 300 degrees. Coat baking sheet with cold-pressed olive oil.

Cut cauliflower into medium-sized florets. Cook in steamer basket over simmering water in covered saucepan for 5–10 minutes or until tender. Remove.

Meanwhile, beat together eggs and sea salt in a mixing bowl. Toss breadcrumbs, basil, and parsley in another mixing bowl. Place flour in bag. Add florets in batches, shaking to coat. Dip florets in egg mixture, then in crumb mixture, turning to coat. Place on prepared baking sheet. Drizzle with butter.

Bake for 30 minutes or until golden and crispy. Serve hot.

Hearty Lentil Loaf (*V) (serves 4–6)
2 cups rinsed lentils
1 bay leaf
1 cup uncooked fine bulgur wheat
1 cup soft whole-wheat bread crumbs
1 egg, beaten
1 T. tomato paste
1 medium onion, chopped
1 clove garlic, crushed
1 t. dried and crumbled thyme
1 t. dried and crumbled tarragon
1 t. sea salt
3 T. tomato paste or tomato sauce
2 t. dried and crumbled oregano

Preheat oven to 350 degrees. Combine lentils and bay leaf in a saucepan with 6 cups water. Bring to a boil, reduce heat, cover, and simmer until lentils are soft and most of the water has been absorbed, about 45 minutes.

Combine bulgur and 2 cups water in a medium saucepan. Bring to a boil, reduce heat, cover, and simmer for 15 minutes. Transfer lentils to a large mixing bowl. Add bulgur and remaining ingredients except tomato paste or sauce. Mix well with your hands until thoroughly combined. Pat mixture into a 9-inch loaf pan. Bake for 40 minutes until firm, but not dry. During the last 5 minutes of baking, brush top with tomato paste or sauce. Let cool for 15 minutes. Cut into slices and serve warm.

Stuffed Cabbage (*V) (serves 6–8)
½ cup uncooked Kasha
½ cup uncooked brown rice mix with wild rice or just brown rice

1 T. curry powder
1 t. ground ginger
1 t. savory
1 t. sea salt
1 T. cold-pressed olive oil
1 cup finely chopped mushrooms
1 small onion, chopped
3 large heads of cabbage
¼ cup currants
½ cup cubed pineapple (canned or fresh)

Preheat oven to 300 degrees. Cook Kasha and rice separately, then cool. In mixing bowl, blend together all ingredients, including Kasha and rice, except cabbage. Prepare cabbage by steaming heads and then place in cool water. Peel back leaves. Roll ¼-½ cup of mixture in cabbage leaf with the large part of the stem rolling forward. Bake for 45 minutes.

Sweet and Sour Tempeh (*V) (serves 6)
½ cup almonds
2 12-oz. blocks tempeh
4 T. tamari
1 large onion
1 each large green and red bell pepper
1 stalk celery
1 large carrot
1 cup fresh pineapple chunks
1 ½ T. honey
2 T. apple cider vinegar
1 ¼ cups vegetable stock or water
1 ½ T. arrowroot

Toast almond pieces in a dry skillet over medium heat and set aside.

Cut tempeh into 2-inch cubes and marinate in 2 T. tamari. Cut onion across center and down into wedge-shaped slices. Cut green pepper in pointy wedges and celery and carrots in thin diagonal slices. Stir-fry in water until crisp tender. Add pineapple after 2–3 minutes.

Combine honey, vinegar, and 1 cup of the vegetable stock, and add to vegetables along with tempeh. Dissolve arrowroot in remaining ¼ cup stock and the remaining 2 T. tamari. Add arrowroot mixture to vegetables to thicken sauce. Cook for 3-4 minutes more. Serve with brown rice.

Tofu Enchiladas (*V) (serves 4-6)
Preheat oven to 350 degrees
Sauce
1 cup tomato sauce
¼ cup chopped onion
1 T. chili powder
1 T. garlic
1 T. cumin
1 T. apple cider vinegar
1 t. Vege Sal
1 T. Spike

Blend in a blender until smooth. Heat and reserve.

Enchilada Mix
14 oz. tofu, crumbled
½ large carrot, chopped
1 stalk celery, chopped
½ squash (any kind), chopped
½ onion, chopped
¼ cauliflower, chopped
1 T. oregano
1 T. cumin
1 t. Vege Sal
6 whole-wheat tortillas

Combine enchilada mix and roll mixture into whole-wheat tortillas. Line enchiladas in a baking dish, top with enchilada sauce, and bake for 30 minutes.

Eggplant Tabouli (*V) (serves 4–6)
1 eggplant sliced thinly, the long way
Olive oil
Sea salt
1 cup couscous
1 cup hot vegetable broth
2 Roma tomatoes, diced
¼ leek, julienne
2 T. chopped basil

Preheat oven to 400 degrees. Lightly brush a cookie sheet with olive oil. Place eggplant on greased cookie sheet. Lightly brush eggplant with olive oil. Sprinkle eggplant with sea salt. Roast eggplant in oven for 5–8 minutes or until supple.

Lightly brush an oven-proof bowl with olive oil, and drape eggplant over sides and in bottom of bowl.

Heat vegetable broth to the boiling point. Pour hot broth over couscous. Stir in basil, tomatoes, and leek. Pour couscous mixture into eggplant "bowl" and cover top with more eggplant.

Reduce heat in oven to 350 degrees and bake for 15 minutes. Turn out onto a plate, cut like a pie, and serve.

Black Bean Soup (*V) (serves 4–6)
½ cup black beans
4 cups water
1 quart soup stock
1 leek, chopped
1 carrot, chopped
2 stalks celery, chopped
1 15-oz. can diced tomatoes
2 T. tomato paste
1 T. chopped garlic
Sea salt to taste
Chopped cilantro for garnish

Soak beans in 4 cups water overnight. Discard water.

In a soup pot, sauté all veggies except tomato products in a little bit of water. When veggies are slightly tender, add soup stock and beans and simmer, stirring occasionally. When beans are tender, add tomato products and continue to simmer 20 minutes. Serve with cilantro garnish.

Spinach Soufflé (*V) (serves 8)
1 whole red onion, chopped
6 egg whites, beaten
3 whole eggs, beaten
1–2 bunches uncooked spinach, chopped medium in food processor
2 cups chopped mushrooms

7 slices whole-grain bread, chopped into medium-sized breadcrumbs
1 cup cashews or Brazilian nuts, chopped fine in food processor
1 T. ground basil
1 T. garlic, chopped fine
⅔ cup tamari
1 t. ground thyme
1 T. lemon juice
½ cup olive oil

Combine and sauté in oil, mushrooms, thyme, basil, lemon juice, and garlic.

In large mixing bowl, combine sautéed mixture, tamari, whole eggs, onion, spinach, bread crumbs, and cashews.

Mix, by hand, and fold in egg whites. Place mixture in 2-inch buttered baking dish. Bake at 350 degrees for 45 minutes.

Mixed Grain & Nut Pilaf (*V) (serves 4–6)
2 cups brown rice
½ cup wild rice
½ cup chopped nuts
2 cups finely chopped mushrooms
1 cup finely chopped red onion
½ cup finely chopped celery
3 T. Braggs
Water as needed

Sauté mushrooms, onion, celery, and wild rice until the veggies are tender. Add these to the remaining ingredients except the water. Place in casserole dish and spread the mixture out evenly. Add the water to the dish so you cover the rice by ½ inch, and place uncovered in the oven at 350 degrees. Check after 30 minutes to see if you need to add water. The wild rice takes longer to cook, so sample it to test for doneness.

Lima Bean Casserole (*V) (serves 4–6)
6 cups lima beans (soaked and cooked) and reserve liquid
3 cups Roma tomatoes, seeded and chopped
3 cups baby spinach
1 cup soy Parmesan cheese
2 T. garlic, chopped

Unrefined sea salt to taste

Bread Crumb Mixture:
3 cups whole-grain bread crumbs
¼ cup chopped thyme
¼ cup chopped Italian parsley
1 stick butter, melted
½ cup grated soy cheese (optional)

Mix the first group of ingredients and taste. If you like it, place the mixture in an uncovered casserole dish. Bake slowly at 275–300 degrees, letting the juices absorb into the beans. Adjust liquid as needed to avoid drying or becoming too much like soup. Top with bread-crumb mixture 20 minutes before the casserole is finished. Let rest for 15 minutes before serving so that the beans will soak up the extra juice.

Eggplant Casserole (*V) (serves 4-6)
2 cups pared and cubed eggplant
1 cup tomato sauce
½ cup chopped green pepper
1 cup chopped onion
2 cups whole-grain bread crumbs
1 t. sea salt
1 T. oregano
1 T. basil
1 t. thyme
1 T. nutmeg
1 t. chopped fresh garlic
1 cup soy cheese, grated

Combine all ingredients (except soy cheese) and pour into casserole dish. Bake in oven at 350 degrees for 45 minutes. Sprinkle soy cheese on top of casserole and bake another 15 minutes.

Appendix Section 4

Rotation Diet

Menu Suggestions for Four-Day Rotation Diet

Day 1:

Breakfast: Cereal—Pearl barley or kamut, walnuts, goat yogurt, and banana, kiwi, or papaya
Green blender drink—Blend romaine lettuce, goat yogurt, pecans or walnuts, and banana, kiwi, or papaya

Lunch: Sautéed mahi-mahi or ahi seasoned with ginger and turmeric
Asparagus with walnut oil, chopped walnuts
Salad of lettuce, chopped bell pepper and jicama, chopped kiwi or papaya, pecans

Dinner: Tuna salad with chopped pecans or walnuts, jicama, and bell pepper

Day 2:

Breakfast: Cereal—Buckwheat or teff, grape or mango, nuts, yogurt
Green blender drink—Kale, mango, blueberries or grapes, yogurt, Brazil nuts

Lunch: Roast turkey with cranberry sauce and gravy or sautéed red snapper or buffalo patties
Steamed broccoli and cauliflower; red cabbage seasoned with vinegar, allspice, and cloves; or steamed Brussels sprouts
Salad of watercress, mangos or grapes, cashews or pistachios

Dinner: Turkey soup with pureed leftover vegetables

Day 3:

Breakfast: Cereal—Spelt or quinoa, berries, sheep yogurt, hazelnuts or pine nuts

Green blender drink—Spinach or chard, berries, sheep yogurt, hazelnuts

Lunch: Lamb patties with sheep yogurt/cumin sauce and mint; sautéed halibut; or sole seasoned with cumin or coriander

Peas, beans, or snow peas with sesame oil

Spinach salad with blackberries, peas, nuts

Dinner: Bean soup with leftover or frozen vegetables

Day 4:

Breakfast: Steel-cut oatmeal or mahogany rice, peaches, soy milk, almonds

Lunch: Meatloaf with grated zucchini and carrots and gravy or sautéed salmon

Steamed carrots, fennel, zucchini squash, or acorn squash with coconut oil, nutmeg

Grated zucchini, carrots, fennel, coconut, chopped almonds

Dinner: Meatloaf wrap with grated zucchini, carrots, fennel in rice tortilla

Recipes for Four-Day Rotation Diet
(All recipes serve 2 people)

Day 1
Breakfast:

Dressed-Up Barley Hot (or Cold) Cereal
½ cup pearl barley
1 cup water
Goat yogurt
Pineapple, banana, or papaya
Walnuts, pecans, or macadamias

Combine barley and water the night before. In the morning, bring to a boil. Simmer 15 minutes. (May also be cooked the same day by combining 1 ½ cups water and ½ cup barley. Bring to a boil and simmer 35–40 minutes. If you have an early-morning rush, grains may be cooked the night before or up to a week ahead and refrigerated. All cooked cereals are good cold too.) Serve with walnuts, pecans, macadamias, diced pineapple, sliced banana, papaya, goat yogurt, as desired. Other grains for this day are kamut and milo, which can be prepared according to producer's instructions and served as above.

Pineapple/Banana Breakfast Smoothie
1 cup pineapple (or 1 banana or both)
4–5 large lettuce leaves
2 cups water (can include vegetable cooking water from day before)

Blend all ingredients in a blender and serve. (Best if blended until very smooth with a good blender, such as Vita-Mix.)

Lunch

Sautéed Cod with Walnuts and Shiitake Mushrooms
2 T. walnut or macadamia oil
8–12 oz. cod (mahi-mahi fine)
⅓ cup walnuts (or macadamias or pecans)
2–3 large shiitake mushrooms
1 t. garlic powder or 1–2 cloves crushed garlic
Sea salt

Put oil in small frying pan and heat on medium-low. Add fish and sauté for a few minutes. Add nuts, shiitakes, and seasonings and cook, covered, until fish is flaky (approximately 10–15 minutes). If you are trying to eliminate calories from oil, you can easily poach the fish by substituting 1 cup water for oil and cook on medium-low until flaky. You can also bake the fish at 350 degrees for 20–30 minutes or until flaky.

Herbed Asparagus (from extra foods)

½ bunch asparagus (or okra)
½ cup water
1 T. walnut oil
1 T. vinegar
Oregano or Italian seasoning (optional)
Sea salt

Steam asparagus in water until fork tender. Pour off water and reserve for breakfast smoothies. Rinse asparagus in cold water to halt cooking. Sprinkle other ingredients over asparagus and roll in pan to coat.

Baked Sweet Potato

1 large sweet potato

Thoroughly wash a sweet potato. Cut off both ends and split down the middle. Place in covered baking dish. Bake at 350 degrees until fork tender, approximately one hour. (You may coat outside of skin with coconut oil prior to cooking for nice flavor.)

Romaine Salad with Pineapple, Jicama, and Pecans

4–5 leaves romaine (or other lettuce)
¼ diced jicama
½ diced pineapple (or apple or pear)
1 T. walnut oil
1 T. ++vinegar
¼ cup pecans (or walnuts)

Chill all ingredients in covered salad bowl. (You can store oil and vinegar in bottom of bowl, under salad until ready to toss. If tossed too soon before serving, greens will wilt.) Toss just before serving.

Dinner:

Tuna Salad with Pineapple, Walnuts, and Jicama
1 can tuna
2 T. mayonnaise
1 T. vinegar
1 clove crushed fresh garlic or garlic powder
Sea salt
4 cups (or more) chopped lettuce
½ diced pineapple (and/or apple, pear, kiwi)
¼ diced jicama
⅓ cup walnuts

Mix tuna with mayo (can substitute oil if necessary) and seasonings. Place lettuce in individual bowls and garnish with pineapple, jicama, and walnuts. Place a scoop of tuna on each salad.

Day 2
Breakfast:

Fancy Teff Breakfast Cereal
½ cup teff (or buckwheat)
1 cup water
Nonfat plain cow yogurt (optional)
Mangos, grapes, blueberries
Pistachios, cashews, Brazil nuts

Combine ingredients in saucepan. Bring to boil. Simmer 15–20 minutes. (Teff will then need to be stirred, since it tends to separate at first.) Serve with diced mango, grapes, cow yogurt, pistachios, cashews, and/or Brazil nuts. (Blueberries may be used for any fruits today and provide great nutrition!) Buckwheat also makes a nice cereal.

Mango-Grape Kale Breakfast Smoothie
4–5 medium kale leaves
1 peeled, coarsely chopped mango and/or 1 cup grapes

Blend until smooth and serve.

Lunch:

Turkey Sauerkraut Melt
2 slices rye bread
Coarsely ground mustard
1 cup sauerkraut
3–4 turkey dogs (or 1 ½ cups sliced turkey)
4 slices cashew cheese or mozzarella (optional)

Preheat oven to 350 degrees. In a greased baking dish, place the two slices of rye bread. Spread coarsely ground mustard over each slice. Place half of sauerkraut on each slice. Place turkey dogs (split down middle) on sauerkraut. Top with slices of cheese. Bake for 20 minutes until hot or cheese is melted.

Steamed Broccoli and Cauliflower
1 small broccoli crown
¼ small head cauliflower
1 cup water
Sea salt
Cashews or pistachios, optional

Clean broccoli and cauliflower and cut into florets. Place in saucepan with water. Bring to boil on medium. Reduce heat and steam 10 minutes or until fork tender. Do not overcook, or vegetables lose color and nutrients. Season with sea salt to taste. Garnish with cashews or pistachios.

Steamed Spicy Cabbage
¼ head red cabbage
1 cup water
Sea salt
¼ t. cinnamon
1 T. vinegar

Clean cabbage and thinly slice. Place in pan with water and bring to a boil. Simmer 10 minutes or until fork tender. Reserve water for breakfast smoothies. Season with sea salt, cinnamon, and vinegar.

Dinner:

Arugula, Mango, and Cashew Salad
4 cups arugula (or watercress)
½ mango, peeled and diced
¼ cup cashews
1 T. canola oil
1 T. vinegar

Clean arugula and place in salad bowl. Garnish with mango and cashews. Chill. Just before serving, toss with oil and vinegar.

Turkey and Cheese Wraps
4 slices roasted turkey
4 slices cashew cheese or mozzarella
2 whole-wheat tortillas
Stone-ground mustard
1 cup arugula
½ cup diced mango or ½ cup grapes
½ cup cashews
Sea salt

Heat griddle or frying pan dry on medium heat. Warm tortillas to soften. Spread each with stone-ground mustard. On each tortilla place 2 slices turkey, 2 slices cheese, ½ cup arugula, ½ of mango or grapes, and ½ of cashews. Season with sea salt. Roll up burrito style. Can be eaten with knife and fork or wrapped in napkin.

or

Buffalo Patty Melts
2 buffalo patties
4 slices provolone (or other cheese)
2 slices rye bread
Stone-ground mustard

Sauté patties in frying pan until brown. Melt cheese on top. Serve on rye bread, spread with mustard. Great with sauerkraut or leftover steamed vegetables.

Day 3
Breakfast:

Quinoa Hot Cereal with Berries and Sheep Yogurt
½ cup quinoa
1 cup water
Berries, diced apple, or diced pear
Pine nuts, sesame seeds, or peanuts
Sheep yogurt

Place quinoa and water in saucepan. Bring to a boil. Reduce heat and simmer 15–20 minutes. Serve with any combination of berries, diced apple, diced pear, pine nuts, sesame seeds, peanuts, and sheep yogurt.

Green Magic Smoothie
4 large chard leaves
2 cups water
1 apple, cored (or 1 cup strawberries or raspberries)

Blend until smooth and serve. Delicious!

Lunch:

Sautéed Filet of Sole with Parsley and Sesame Seeds
8–12 oz. filet of sole
2 T. olive oil
Parsley
Sesame seeds

Heat olive oil in sauté pan on medium heat. Add filet of sole, lower heat, and cook, covered, until flaky. (This fish cooks very quickly.) Garnish with parsley and sesame seeds. (This recipe is great with mushrooms added to the sauté, if you haven't had them in four days.)

or

Lamb Patties with Dill Sauce for Main Dish or Wrap
½ lb. ground lamb
1 clove crushed garlic
⅛ t. cayenne pepper

⅛ t. fennel seed
⅛ t. cinnamon
⅛ t. cumin seed
⅛ t. coriander seed
⅛ t. oregano
Sea salt
½ cup sheep yogurt
½ t. dill weed

Preheat oven to 350 degrees. Thoroughly mix lamb, garlic, and spices in a bowl with clean hands. Shape into two patties. Place in baking dish uncovered. Bake 20 minutes or until desired doneness is reached. (Juices will run over down the edges when thoroughly cooked.) Season cooked patties with sea salt. Mix yogurt and dill weed and serve as sauce over the top. (I usually mix the spices in a larger quantity, such as 2 t. of each and keep in a jar. Then all I have to do is add ¾ teaspoon of the mixture to the lamb.)

These patties can be served with vegetables or in a wrap. For the wrap, place on a warmed tortilla 1 sliced lamb patty, 2–3 T. yogurt sauce, a handful of pine nuts, and some spinach leaves. Season with salt and wrap up. Delicious!

Snow Pea Pods and Garden Peas
20 snow pea pods
½ cup frozen peas
½ cup water
Sea salt

Place pea pods, peas, and water in saucepan. Bring to boil over medium heat. Simmer approximately 5 minutes or until fork tender. Season with sea salt.

Beautiful Beets
2 small beets
1 cup water
Sea salt

Wash, peel, and quarter beets. Put in saucepan with water. Boil 15 minutes or until fork tender. Season with sea salt.

Tasty Beet Greens
1 bunch beet greens
1 T. vinegar

1 T. sesame oil
1 cup water
Sea salt
Sesame seeds

Thoroughly wash greens and stems. Slice across greens and stems in ½-inch strips. Place in pan with water. Bring to a boil over medium heat. Simmer 5 minutes or until wilted. Pour off water and reserve for breakfast drink. Season with vinegar, oil, and sea salt. Garnish with sesame seeds.

Strawberry and Spinach Salad with Pine Nuts

2 cups spinach
½ cup sliced strawberries (or raspberries)
⅓ cup pine nuts
1 T. olive oil
2 T. vinegar (balsamic, rice wine, red wine, etc.)

Place spinach in salad bowl. Garnish with berries and pine nuts. Chill. Before serving, toss with oil and vinegar.

Dinner:

Easy Guacamole

1 mashed avocado
2 T. salsa (check ingredients)
Sea salt
Juice of ½ orange (optional)
Juice of ½ lemon (optional)
2 T. onion (optional)

Mix all ingredients and serve with eggs.

Apple Wedges with Tahini

2 apples, cut in wedges
4 T. tahini (sesame butter) or peanut butter

Serve apple wedges with tahini as a side dish or snack.

Easy Old-Fashioned Cinnamon Apple Sauce
2 apples
½ t. cinnamon
1 cup water

Thinly slice peeled apples and place in saucepan with water. Simmer until mushy. Break up with spoon or potato masher. Season with cinnamon.

Day 4
Breakfast:

Whole-Grain Oatmeal with Sliced Peaches and Sunflower Seeds
½ cup whole-grain or steel-cut oats
1 ½ cups water
Peaches, apricots, nectarines, cherries, or plums
Almonds, Sunflower (or pumpkin seeds)

Place oats and water in saucepan. Bring to boil. Simmer 50–60 minutes. Serve with sliced peaches, apricots, nectarines, cherries, or plums and almonds, sunflower or pumpkin seeds, or any combination of these that you like.

Melon Slush Smoothie
½ cantaloupe with rind and seeds removed
1 stalk fennel, with leaves
1 large stalk celery or equivalent celery leaves
2 cups water
⅓ cup baby carrots

Blend all ingredients until smooth and serve. This recipe is also delicious with watermelon as a substitute for the cantaloupe. We also like to use beet juice from previous day for part of the water. This really makes a beautiful color!

Lunch:

Sautéed Salmon with Capers and Stone-Ground Mustard
8–12 oz. wild salmon
2 T. coconut oil
2 T. stone-ground mustard
Sea salt
1 T. capers

Heat oil in sauté pan. Add salmon and cook, covered, on medium-low until flaky, about 10 minutes. Top with mustard/caper mixture.

Coconut, Carrot, Squash Slaw
1 small zucchini, grated
1 small crooked-neck squash, grated
1 large carrot, grated
¼ cup grated unsweetened coconut
½ cup soaked almonds
2 T. vinegar
¼ t. stevia
2 T. almond oil

Combine all ingredients and chill until ready to serve.

Steamed Parsnips, Carrots, and Squash
1 parsnip, peeled and sliced
1 small zucchini, sliced
1 small crooked-neck squash, sliced
1 cup baby carrots
1 cup water
Sea salt

Place all ingredients in saucepan. Bring to a boil. Reduce to simmer and cook approximately 10 minutes or until fork tender. Season with sea salt before serving.

Dinner:

Salmon Quesadillas
1 can good quality salmon
4 slices soy cheese (optional)
2 rice tortillas
Olive or Coconut oil

Lightly grease an iron grill or heavy frying pan with coconut or olive oil. Open salmon and mash in bowl until thoroughly mixed. On medium heat, grill warm tortilla to soften. Fill with half of salmon and half of soy cheese. Fold in half and place on grill, lightly covered with flat lid. Cook on medium until lightly browned. Flip over and brown the other side. You can cook 2 quesadillas at once.

Celery Sticks with Almond Butter
3 large stalks celery, sliced lengthwise and cut into 2-inch lengths
4 T. almond butter

After cutting, chill celery in covered container until ready to serve. Serve with almond butter. My husband calls this his dessert!

Rotation Diet
Example of 4-Day Rotation

FOOD GROUPS	DAY ONE	DAY TWO	DAY THREE	DAY FOUR
Protein: Meat/Fish/ Poultry	Turkey, pheasant, chicken, Cornish hen, quail, duck, goose, ostrich, grouse, partridge, eggs of birds, herring, sardine, snapper (red and other types) anchovy, scallops	Beef, buffalo, moose, venison, oysters, clams, crab, lobster, crayfish, shrimp, mussels	Rabbit, cod, haddock, ocean perch, Albacore tuna, mackerel, flounder, sole, turbot, marlin, bass, catfish, eel	Pork, goat, lamb, salmon, trout, smelt, whitefish, perch, walleye, pike, pickerel, snails, squid, octopus
Nuts/Seeds	Hazelnuts, pine nuts, sunflower seeds, macadamia nuts, chestnuts	Pumpkin seeds, poppy seeds acorn, almonds	Walnut, pecan, hickory, peanut, cashew, pistachio caraway seed, sesame seed	Brazil nut, litchi nut, psyllium seeds, coconut, flax seeds
Grains/Starchy Vegetables	Buckwheat, artichoke, lotus, chestnut (starch, flour, bread & pastas) Arrowroot, Malanga (oriental potato or eddoes), tapioca, cassava	Rice, wild rice, corn, millet, teff, job's tears (flour, breads & pastas)	Soy, lentil, chickpea, carob, kudzu, guar gum, water chestnut, quinoa, amaranth, yam (flour, breads & pastas)	Wheat, oats, rye, barley, spelt, kamut, sago, flax (flour, breads & pastas)
Vegetables	Potato, tomato, eggplant, green/ yellow/red peppers, artichoke, lettuce (Boston or romaine, etc.), endive, radicchio	Cucumber, squash, pumpkin, zucchini, asparagus, onion, garlic, leek, chives, shallots, bamboo shoots	Peas, beans, carob, soy, tofu, alfalfa, carrot, celery, parsley, fennel, parsnip, green/ black olives, plantain, water chestnuts, yam, sweet potato, spinach, beets, Swiss chard	Cabbage, cauliflower, broccoli, Brussels sprouts, radish, turnip, rutabaga, rapini, collards, kale, kohlrabi, bok choy, cress, arugula, okra, yucca, mushroom, yeast
Fruit	Strawberry, raspberry, blackberry, boysenberry, rhubarb, blueberry, cranberry, huckleberry	Cantaloupe, casaba, honey dew, watermelon, apricot, cherry, chokecherry, peach, prune, nectarine, plum, avocado	Mango, gooseberry, currants, banana, orange, lemon, lime, grapefruit, tangerine, uglifruit, kumquat, guava, persimmon, fig, mulberry, breadfruit	Grape, raisin, pineapple, pomegranate, kiwi, papaya, apple, pear, quince, cabbage, dates

Herbs/Spices/ Etc.	Paprika, juniper, wintergreen, tarragon, salsify, mint, oregano, sage, thyme, allspice, basil, savory, rosemary, chocolate, black pepper	Lemon grass, poppy seed, capers, clove, allspice, bay leaf, cinnamon, almond extract	Anise, caraway, chervil, coriander, cumin, dill, fennel, ginger, cardamom, turmeric, nutmeg, mace, carob, tamarind	Paprika, cream of tartar, mustard, horseradish, vanilla
Beverages	Potato milk, teas (chamomile, chicory, mint, spearmint, peppermint), cranberry juice	Teas (cinnamon, sassafras or aloe vera), almond milk, rice milk, cow's milk, coffee	Teas (ginger or alfalfa), soya milk, cashew milk, orange juice, lemonade, apricot juice, peach juice, prune juice	Teas (rose hip, vanilla, black or green), papaya juice, grape juice, apple juice, pineapple juice, coconut milk, goat milk
Oils/Fats	Sunflower oil, safflower oil	Almond oil, hemp oil	Sesame oil, olive oil	Canola oil, flax oil, coconut oil
Snacks	Potato chips, sunflower seeds	Corn chips, popcorn, rice crackers	Carob bars, soya nuts, sesame seeds	Dates, raisins, granola
Sweetener	Stevia, frozen concentrated raspberry or cranberry juice	Rice syrup, molasses	Maple sugar or syrup, frozen concentrated citrus juices	Kiwi sweetener, frozen pineapple, apple or grape juice, honey, date sugar

Helpful Hints for Rotation Diet

1. Modify the grocery list attached to fit your plan. Store staples such as seeds, nuts, nut butters, oils, grains, flours, breads (freeze), and frozen fruits/vegetables to have on hand. When shopping, stick to whole, unprocessed foods to avoid allergenic ingredients.

2. Organize refrigerator and freezer and label shelves 1, 2, 3, and 4 for each day. This makes it easier to find what you and family members can eat on that day.

3. Each day, check for ingredients needed for the following day and defrost as needed.

4. All cooking for each day can be done at one time by preparing fruits, vegetables, salad, etc. and refrigerating on shelf for that day.

5. Use masking tape and marking pen to label refrigerator and freezer dishes with 1, 2, 3, or 4 and name of food.

Grocery List

VEGETABLES
- ❑—Asparagus-1
- ❑—Arugula-2
- ❑—Artichoke-1
- ❑—Avocado-3
- ❑—Beans-3
- ❑—Beets-3
- ❑—Broccoli-2
- ❑—Brussels Sprouts-2
- ❑—Cabbage-2
- ❑—Carrots-4
- ❑—Cauliflower-2
- ❑—Celery-4
- ❑—Chard-3
- ❑—Cucumbers-4
- ❑—Endive-1
- ❑—Fennel-4
- ❑—Jicama-1
- ❑—Kale-2
- ❑—Lettuce-1
- ❑—Mushrooms
- ❑—Okra-1
- ❑—Parsley-4
- ❑—Parsnips-4
- ❑—Peppers-1
- ❑—Radicchio-1
- ❑—Potatoes-1
- ❑—Pumpkin-4
- ❑—Romaine-1
- ❑—Squash-4
- ❑—Spinach-3
- ❑—Watercress-2
- ❑—Zucchini-4

FRUITS
- ❑—Apples-3
- ❑—Apricots-4
- ❑—Bananas-1

- ❑—Berries-3
- ❑—Cherries-4
- ❑—Figs-2
- ❑—Grapefruit-3
- ❑—Grapes-2
- ❑—Kiwi-1
- ❑—Lemons-3
- ❑—Limes-3
- ❑—Mango-2
- ❑—Melon-4
- ❑—Oranges-3
- ❑—Nectarines-4
- ❑—Papaya-1
- ❑—Peaches-4
- ❑—Pears-3
- ❑—Persimmons-1
- ❑—Pineapple-1
- ❑—Plums-4
- ❑—Tangerines-3

GRAINS/NUTS
- ❑—Almonds-4
- ❑—Amaranth-1
- ❑—Barley-1
- ❑—Beans-3
- ❑—Brazil Nuts-2
- ❑—Buckwheat-2
- ❑—Cashews-2
- ❑—Filberts-3
- ❑—Hazelnuts-3
- ❑—Kamut-1
- ❑—Lentils-3
- ❑—Macadamia-1
- ❑—Millet-3
- ❑—Oats-4
- ❑—Peanuts-3
- ❑—Pecans-1
- ❑—Pine Nuts-3

- ❑—Pistachios-2
- ❑—Pumpkin Seeds-4
- ❑—Quinoa-3
- ❑—Rice-4
- ❑—Rye-2
- ❑—Sesame Seeds-3
- ❑—Spelt-3
- ❑—Split Peas-3
- ❑—Sunflower-4
- ❑—Teff-2
- ❑—Walnuts-1
- ❑—Wheat-3

DAIRY
- ❑—Butter-2
- ❑—Cow Yogurt-2
- ❑—Eggs-3
- ❑—Goat Yogurt-1
- ❑—Sheep Yogurt-3

CHEESES
- ❑—Cow-2
- ❑—Cream-2
- ❑—Goat-1
- ❑—Sheep-3
- ❑—Soy-4

**MEAT, FISH &
POULTRY**
- ❑—Ahi/Tuna-1
- ❑—Beef-4
- ❑—Buffalo-2
- ❑—Halibut-3
- ❑—Lamb-3
- ❑—Mahi-1
- ❑—Orange Roughy-4
- ❑—Pork-1
- ❑—Red Snapper-2

❑—Salmon-4
❑—Sea Bass-2
❑—Sole-3
❑—Turkey-2

CONDIMENTS
❑—Almond Oil-4
❑—Almond Butter-4
❑—Canola Oil-2
❑—Cashew Butter-2
❑—Coconut Oil-4
❑—Grapeseed Oil-2
❑—Mayonnaise
❑—Macademia
     Butter-1
❑—Mustard-2
❑—Olive Oil-3
❑—Palm Oil-1
❑—Peanut Butter-3
❑—Safflower Oil-1
❑—Sesame Oil-3
❑—Sunflower Oil-4
❑—Tamari-4
❑—Walnut Oil-1

Information on Food Families
Food Families Index

The food families index lists the botanical family for most common foods. If you reacted to more than two members of the same food family, there is a possibility that other members of that family may be a source of symptoms. Refer to the food families to identify additional members. Please avoid these additional foods if you develop symptoms when you eat them.

Foods	Family	Foods	Family
Alfalfa	Legume	Cashew	Cashew
Almond	Rose	Cauliflower	Mustard
Avocado	Laurel	Celery	Carrot
Amaranth	Pursuance	Cheese	Bovine/Fungus
Apple	Rose	Cherry	Rose
Asparagus	Lily	Chicken	Pheasant
Baker's Yeast	Fungus	Chili Pepper	Nightshade
Banana	Banana	Cinnamon	Laurel
Barley	Grass	Clam	Mollusk
Mint	Mint	Clove	Myrtle
Beef	Bovine	Cocoa-Chocolate	Specula
Beet	Goosefoot	Coconut	Palm
Black Pepper	Pepper	Cod	Codfish
Brazil Nut	Sapodilla	Coffee	Madder
Brewer's Yeast	Fungus	Corn	Grain/Grasses
Broccoli	Mustard	Cow's Milk	Bovine
Brussels Sprouts	Mustard	Crab	Crustacean
Buckwheat	Buckwheat	Cranberry	Heath
Cabbage	Mustard	Egg	Pheasant
Cane Sugar	Grain/Grass	Eggplant	Nightshade
Cantaloupe	Gourd	Flounder	Flounder
Carrot	Carrot	Garlic	Lily
Ginger	Ginger	Parsley	Carrot
Goat's Milk	Bovine	Pea	Legume
Grape	Grape	Peach	Rose
Grapefruit	Citrus	Peanut	Legume
Green Beans	Legume	Pecan	Walnut
Green Pepper	Nightshade	Perch	Bass

Foods	Family	Foods	Family
Haddock	Cod	Pineapple	Pineapple
Halibut	Flounder	Pinto Bean	Legume
Herring	Herring	Plum	Rose
Kidney	Legume	Pork	Swine
Lamb	Bovine	Pumpkin	Gourd
Lemon	Citrus	Quinoa	Goosefoot
Lentil	Legume	Radish	Mustard
Lettuce	Composite	Rape Seed (canola)	Mustard
Lima Bean	Legume	Rice	Grain/Grass
Lime	Citrus	Rye	Grain/Grass
Lobster	Crustacean	Safflower	Composite
Mackerel	Mackerel	Sage	Mint
Millet	Grass	Salmon	Salmon
Mung Bean Sprouts	Legume	Scallop	Mollusk
Mushroom	Fungus	Sesame	Pendulum
Mustard	Mustard	Shrimp	Crustacean
Nutmeg	Nutmeg	Snapper	Bass
Oat	Grass	Sole	Flounder
Olive	Olive	Soybean	Legume
Onion	Lily	Spinach	Goosefoot
Orange	Citrus	Strawberry	Rose
Oregano	Mint	Sunflower	Composite
Oyster	Mollusk	Sweet Potato	Morning Glory
Papaya	Papaya	Tangerine	Citrus
Tea	Tea	Whitefish	Salmon
Tomato	Nightshade	White Pepper	Pepper
Trout	Salmon	White Potato	Nightshade
Tuna	Mackerel	Yam	Yam
Turkey	Turkey	Yellow Wax Beans	Legume
Walnut	Walnut	Zucchini	Gourd
Wheat	Grain/Grasses		

Food Families

Plant

Algae
Agar
Carrageen (Irish moss)
Dulles
Kelp

Amaranth Family
Amaranth
Quinoa

Amaryllis Family
Agaves
Mescal, pique
Tequila

Arum Family
Ceriman
    dasheen (white yam)
    mélange arrowroot
    taro
    arrowroot
    poi

Banana Family
Arrowroot (muse)
Banana
Plantain

Beech Family
Chestnut
Chinquapin

Birch Family
Filbert (hazelnut)
Oil of birch
(wintergreen)

(some wintergreen
flavor is methyl
calculate)

Bexar Family
Annatto (natural
yellow dye)
Borage Family
Borage
Comfrey (leaf & root)

Buckwheat Family
Buckwheat
Garden sorrel
Rhubarb
Sea grape

Buttercup Family
Golden seal

Cactus Family
Prickly pear

Cannas Family
Queensland arrowroot

Caper Family
Caper

Carpetweed Family
New Zealand spinach

Carrot Family
Angelica
Anise
Caraway
Carrot
Celeriac (celery root)

Celery (seed & leaf)
Chervil
Coriander
Cumin
Dill
Dill seed
Fennel
Pinocchio
Florence fennel
Gout kola
Lesage
Parsley
Parsnip
Sweet cicely

Cashew Family
Cashew
Mango
Pistachio
Poison ivy
Poison oak
Poison sumac

Composite Family
Boneset
Burdock root
Cardoon
Chamomile
Chicory
Coltsfoot
Costmary
Dandelion
Endive
Escarole
Globe artichoke
Jerusalem artichoke
Lettuce
Celtic

Pyrethrum
Romaine
Safflower oil
Falsify (oyster plant)
Semolina (herb)
Columbus (Spanish oyster plant)
Coroner (black falsify)
Southernwood
Sunflower (seed, meal, oil, butter)
Tansy (herb)
Tarragon (herb)
Wit off chicory (French endive)
Wormwood (absinthe)
Yarrow

Conifer Family
Juniper (gin)
Pine nut

Custard-Apple Family
Cherimoya
Custard-apple
Pawpaw

Cycad Family
Florida arrowroot (zamia)

Ebony Family
American persimmon
Kaki (Japanese persimmon)

Flax Family
Flaxseed

Fungi Family
Baker's yeast ("Red Star")
Brewer's yeast
Mold (certain cheeses)
Citric acid (aspergillums)
Morel
Mushroom
Puffball
Truffle

Ginger Family
Cardamom
East Indian arrowroot
Ginger
Turmeric

Ginseng family
American ginseng
Chinese ginseng

Goosefoot Family
Beet
Chard
Lamb's quarters
Spinach
Sugar beet
Tambala

Gourd Family
Chayote
Chinese preserving melon
Cucumber
Gherkin
Lora (vegetable sponge)
Muskmelons
    cantaloupe
    casaba
    Crenshaw

honeydew
    Persian melon
Pumpkin (seeds & meal)
Squashes
    acorn
    buttercup
    Boston marrow
    casita
cocozelle
    crookneck
    straightneck
    cushaw
    golden nugget
    hubbard varieties
    pattypan
    turban
    spaghetti
    zucchini
watermelon

Grape Family
Grape
    brandy
    champagne
    cream of tartar
    dried currant
    raisin
    wine
    wine vinegar
Muscadine

Grass Family
Barley
    malt
    maltose
Bamboo shoots
Corn
    cornmeal
    corn oil
    cornstarch

corn sugar
corn syrup
hominy grits
popcorn
Lemon grass
citronella
Millet
Oat
oatmeal
Rice, rice flour
Rye
Teff
Sorghum
Sugar cane
cane sugar
molasses
raw sugar
Sweet corn
Triticale
Wheat
Bran
Bulgur
Wheat germ
Kamut
Wild rice
Spelt
Couscous

Heath Family
Bearberry
Blueberry
Cranberry
Huckleberry

Holly Family
Mate (yerba mate)

Honeysuckle Family
Elderberry
elderberry flowers

Horsetail Family
Shavegrass (horsetail)

Iris Family
Oris root (scent)
Saffron (crocus)

Laurel Family
Avocado
Bay leaf
Cassia bark
Cinnamon
Sassafras
Filé (powdered leaves)

Legume Family
Alfalfa (sprouts)
Beans
fava
lima
mung (sprouts)
navy
string (kidney)
Black-eyed peas
(cowpea)
Carob
carob syrup
Chickpea (garbanzo)
Fenugreek
Gum acacia
Gum tragacanth
Jicama
Kudzu
Lentil
Licorice
Pea
Peanut
Peanut oil
Red clover
Senna
Soybean

lecithin
soy flour
soy grits
soy milk
soy oil
Tamarind
Tonka bean
coumarin

Lily Family
Asparagus
Chives
Garlic
Garlic chives
Leek
Onion
Ramp
Sarsaparilla
Shallot
Yucca (soap plant)

Linden Family
Basswood (linden)

Madder Family
Coffee
Woodruff

Mallow Family
Althea root
Cottonseed oil
Hibiscus (roselle)
Okra

Malpighia Family
Acerola (Barbados
cherry)

Maple Family
Maple sugar
Maple syrup

Millennia Family
Chinese gooseberry
   (kiwi berry)

Mint Family
Apple mint
Basil
Bergamot
Catnip
Chia seed
Clary
Dittany
Horehound
Hyssop
Lavender
Lemon balm
Marjoram
Oregano
Pennyroyal
Peppermint
Rosemary
Sage
Spearmint
Summer savory
Thyme
Winter savory

Morning Glory Family
Camote
Sweet potato

Mulberry Family
Breadfruit
Fig
Hemp
Hop
Mulberry

Mustard Family
Bok choy
Broccoli
Brussels sprouts
Cabbage
Cardoon
Cauliflower
Chinese cabbage
Colza shoots
Collards
Couve tronchuda
Curly cress
Horseradish
Kale
Kohlrabi
Mustard seed
Mustard greens
Napa
Radish
Rape
Rutabaga (swede)
Turnip
Upland cress
Watercress

Myrtle Family
Allspice (pimenta)
Clove
Eucalyptus
Guava

Nasturtium Family
Nasturtium
   seed
   leaf
   flower

Nutmeg Family
Nutmeg
Mace

Olive Family
Olive
   olive oil

Orchid Family
Vanilla

Oxalis Family
Carambola
Oxalis

Palm Family
Coconut
   leaf
   meal
   milk
   oil
   seed
Date
   date sugar
Palm cabbage
Sago starch

Papaya Family
Papaya

Passion Flower Family
Granadilla (passion fruit)

Pedalium Family
Sesame seed
Sesame oil
   tahini

Pepper Family
Peppercorn
   black pepper
   white pepper

Pineapple Family
Pineapple

Pomegranate Family
Pomegranate
Grenadine

Poppy Family
Poppyseed

Potato Family
Eggplant
Ground cherry
Pepino (melon pear)
Pepper (capsicum)
 bell, sweet
 cayenne
 chili
 paprika
 pimiento
Potato
Tobacco
Tomatillo
Tomato
Tree tomato

Protea Family
Macadamia
(Queensland nut)

Purslane Family
Pigweed

Rose Family
Pomes
 apple
 cider
 crabapple
 loquat
 pear

pectin
quince
rosehips
vinegar
Stone Fruits
 almond
 apricot
 cherry
 peach (nectarine)
 plum (prune)
 sloe
Berries
 blackberry
 black raspberry
 boysenberry
 dewberry
 loganberry
 longberry
 purple raspberry
 raspberry (leaf)
 red raspberry
 strawberry (leaf)
 tayberry
 wineberry
 youngberry
Herb
 burnet (cucumber
flavor)

Rue (citrus) Family
Citron
Grapefruit
Kumquat
Lemon
Lime
Murcot
Orange
Pummelo
Tangelo
Tangerine
Ugli fruit

Sapodilla Family
Chicle (chewing gum)

Sapucaya Family
Brazil nut
Sapucaya nut (paradise
nut)

Saxifrage Family
Currant
Gooseberry

Sedge Family
Chinese water chestnut
Chufa (groundnut)

Soapberry Family
Litchi (lychee)

Spurge Family
Cassave or yucca
 cassave meal
Tapioca (Brazilian
arrowroot)
 castor bean

Sterculia Family
Chocolate (cacao)
Cocoa
 cocoa butter
Cola nut

Tacca Family
Fiji arrowroot

Tea Family
Tea

Valerian Family
Corn salad (fetticus)

Verbena Family
Lemon verbena

Walnut Family
Black walnut
Butternut
English walnut
Heartnut
Hican
Hickory nut
Pecan

Yam Family
Chinese potato (yam)
Name (yampi)

Animal

Anchovy Family
Anchovy

Bass Family
Yellow bass

Bear Family
Bear

Bluefish Family
Bluefish

Bovine Family
Beef
Beef byproducts
    gelatin
    oleomargarine
    rennin (rennet)
    sausage casings
    suet
Buffalo (Bison)
Goat
    milk products
Milk products
    butter
    cheese
    ice cream
    lactose
    spray-dried milk
    yogurt
Rocky Mountain sheep
Sheep
    lamb
    mutton
Veal

Catfish Family
Catfish

Codfish Family
Cod (scrod)
Cusk
Haddock
Jake
Pollack

Croaker Family
Croaker
Drum
Sea trout
Silver perch
Spot
Spotted sea trout

Crustaceans
Crab
Crayfish
Lobster
Prawn
Shrimp

Deer Family
Caribou
Deer (venison)
Elk
Moose
Reindeer

Dolphin Family
Dolphin

Dove Family
Dove
Pigeon (squab)

Duck Family
Duck
Duck eggs

Goose
Goose eggs

Eel Family
American eel

Flounder Family
Dab
Flounder
Halibut
Plaice
Sole
Turbot

Frog Family
Frog

Grouse Family
Ruffed grouse
(partridge)

Guinea Fowl Family
Guinea fowl
Guinea fowl eggs

Hare Family
Rabbit

Harvestfish Family
Butterfish
Harvestfish

Herring Family
Menhaden
Pilchard (sardine)
Sea herring
Shad
Sprat

Horse Family
Horse

Jack Family
Amberjack
Pompano
Yellow jack

Mackerel Family
Albacore
Bonito
Mackerel
Skipjack
Tuna

Marlin Family
Marlin
Sailfish

Minnow
Carp
Chub

Mollusks
Gastropods
    abalone
    snail
Cephalopod
    squid
Pelecypods
    clam
    cockle
    mussel
    oyster
    scallop

Mullet Family
Mullet

Opposum Family
Opposum

Perch and Pike Family
Muskellunge
Pickerel
Pike
Sauger (perch)
Walleye
Yellow perch

Pheasant Family
Chicken
Chicken eggs
Peafowl
Pheasant
Quail

Porgy Family
Northern scup (porgy)

Pronghorn Family
Antelope

Ratite Family
Emu
Ostrich
Rhea

Salmon Family
Salmon
Trout

Scorpionfish Family
Rosefish (ocean perch)

Sea Bass Family
Grouper
Sea bass

Sea Catfish Family
Ocean catfish

Silverside Family
Silverside (whitebait)

Smelt Family
Smelt

Snake Family
Rattlesnake

Snapper Family
Red snapper

Squirrel Family
Squirrel

Sturgeon Family
Sturgeon (caviar)

Sucker Family
Buffalofish
Sucker

Sunfish Family
Black bass species
Sunfish species
    pumpkinseed
Crappie

Swine Family
Hog (pork)
    bacon
    ham
    lard
    pork gelatin
    sausage
    scrappie

Swordfish Family
Swordfish

Tilefish Family
Tilefish

Turkey Family
Turkey
Turkey eggs

Turtle Family
Terrapin
Turtle species

Whale Family
Whale

Whitefish Family
Whitefish

Appendix Section 5
Wheat-free Diet

Nancy's High-Fiber Bean and Veggie Burritos (*V) (serves 2)
2 large corn tortillas
Filling:
¾ cup refried beans (vegetarian-style)
1 cup fresh or steamed veggies (carrots, squash, mushrooms, etc.)
¼ cup fresh salsa
¼ cup low-fat sour cream (optional)

Place beans and veggies in tortillas. Combine salsa and sour cream in a blender and blend until smooth. Divide salsa mixture between two tortillas and roll up burrito-style.

Nancy's Cheesy Corn-Pasta Primavera (*V) (serves 2–3)
1 cup cooked corn pasta (available in natural-food stores)
2 cups steamed vegetables (broccoli, cauliflower, etc.)
1 T. olive oil or butter
½ cup cottage cheese (or fat-free soy cheese, grated)
1 t. garlic powder or no-salt garlic blend
4 T. Parmesan cheese (or soy parmesan)

Combine hot cooked pasta with steamed veggies in large bowl. Add oil, cottage cheese, garlic, and only 2 T. of Parmesan cheese into pasta/veggie mix. Top with remaining 2 T. Parmesan. Enjoy!

Soft Rolled Tacos (*V) (serves 2)
Mix the following together in a small bowl:
1 cup fresh tossed mixed greens or sprouts
1 medium carrot, grated
1 small tomato, diced

2 oz. cooked chicken breast, cut into cubes

or

4 oz. baked tofu (available at natural-food stores)
1 recipe Nancy's Fat-Free Spicy Dijon Dressing (blend 4 T. vinegar, ½ T. mustard, and ½ T. honey until creamy or mix in a jar and shake to blend)

2 medium unbaked corn tortillas

Stuff tortillas with filling and dressing taco-style.

Nancy's Oriental Veggie Stir-Fry (*V) (serves 2)
3 oz. chicken, beef, tofu, or shrimp, cut in small pieces
2 cups fresh veggies of choice, chopped in small pieces
1 T. oil or water
1 t. garlic powder
2 T. wheat-free tamari
2 t. sesame seeds

In large pan, combine the oil and garlic powder and meat or tofu and cook until done. Add 2 cups of veggies and tamari and cook until veggies are desired texture. Top with sesame seeds.

Mashed Cauliflower *(A great substitute for mashed potatoes)* (*V) (serves 6)
1 bag frozen cauliflower florets
4–6 oz. cream cheese (to taste)
3 T. whole milk or half & half
Butter (to taste)
Salt/Pepper (to taste)
Garlic salt, ranch dressing powder, pepper, parmesan, etc. for flavor (optional)

Microwave the cauliflower in large glass bowl covered with a plate to keep the steam in. Cook until cauliflower is very well done (soft!) approx. 8–10 minutes. Drain.

When cauliflower is cool enough for you to handle, *squeeze as much water out of it as possible.* Put the cauliflower into a food processor and whir on high just until it gets very smooth. Add only 2 T. of milk, cream cheese, and butter. Mix well. The whole point of this process is to make the cauliflower creamy and smooth. Check the consistency. If it is too thick for you, add a tiny bit of milk, mix, and check again. Too much liquid and you will end up with soup (hence the draining!).

Serve hot/warm; you may need to heat it quickly in the microwave before serving.

For a colorful dish, try adding a small amount of carrots or broccoli with the cauliflower

Confetti Veggie Salsa & Multi-Bean Chili Pie in a Polenta Chili Relleno Pastry Bowl (serves 4–6)

Polenta Chili Relleno Pastry Bowl:
2 cups + 2 T. cornmeal (save 2 T. for dusting pan)
1 cup nonfat milk
2 T. canola or olive oil or melted butter
1 T. honey or fruit juice concentrate
1 large egg or 2 egg whites (beaten slightly)
1 ½ t. baking powder
¼ cup green chilies (canned, mild)
½ cup low-fat cheddar cheese, grated

Confetti Salsa/Chili Filling:
2 T. liquid from drained salsa below
4 cloves fresh garlic, minced
1 cup red onion, diced
1 cup zucchini, diced
1 cup green bell pepper, diced
1 cup corn, frozen or fresh off the cob
½ cup chunky-style salsa (liquid drained)
2 t. cumin
2 t. oregano
3 T. chili powder
1 15-oz. can whole tomatoes, drained
1 15-oz. can black beans, drained and rinsed
1 15-oz. can kidney beans, drained and rinsed
½ lb. cooked veggie burger or ground turkey breast, crumbled (optional)

Topping:
¼ cup fresh cilantro, chopped
1 cup Mexican cotija cheese or low-fat cheddar, grated
½ cup Parmesan cheese, grated

Polenta Chili Relleno Pastry Bowl: Combine milk, oil, and honey in saucepan and warm over medium heat until honey melts, or microwave for 20 seconds. Add cornmeal, baking powder, and egg, and mix to form a sticky dough. Fold in chilies and cheese until well mixed. Spray baking dish with nonstick spray And dust with approx. 2 T. cornmeal. Press dough out evenly to cover pan and make outside edge. Bake at 350 degrees for 15 minutes to seal crust.

Confetti Salsa: In large saucepan, add first 9 ingredients for filling and cook over medium-high heat for 10 minutes until veggies are slightly tender and flavors are released (this can be done a day before and refrigerated for later).

Add the next 4 ingredients to the cooked Confetti Salsa and heat over medium-high until hot throughout (about 15 minutes). Pour Chili/Salsa mix into partially cooked cornmeal pastry bowl, add mixed topping evenly, and bake for 20 to 30 minutes more.

Wheat-Free Sunflower, Millet, and White Corn Enchiladas with a Black Bean and Tomato Garlic Sauce (serves 6–8)
1 cup cooked millet (cook in 2 parts water to 1 part millet until tender)
½ large onion, minced
1 cup white corn, frozen or cut off the cob
¼ cup sunflower seeds (toasted, if desired)
1 t. garlic powder
1 recipe Black Bean and Tomato Garlic Sauce *(follows)*
1 cup low-fat ricotta cheese
1 cup low-fat jack cheese
8 medium corn tortillas
½ cup parmesan cheese
1 can diced green chilies (optional)
1 cup zucchini, shredded (optional)

Preheat oven to 350 degrees. In large skillet add cooked millet plus next 4 ingredients and 1 cup of the black bean tomato sauce plus ½ cup water. Cook over medium heat just until mix is hot. Remove from heat, mix in the ricotta cheese and only ¼ cup parmesan, and add any optional ingredients at this time.

In hot oven, warm tortillas wrapped in foil for 2–3 minutes or microwave for 30 seconds to soften.

To make enchiladas: Spread 1 T. of black bean tomato sauce over warmed tortilla, add ½ cup millet filling, and sprinkle with 2 T. jack cheese. Roll up carefully and fit into 8x8 pan. Cover with remaining sauce and sprinkle with parmesan. Bake until hot throughout, approximately 20 minutes.

Black Bean and Tomato Garlic Sauce (serves 3–4)

4 cloves garlic, minced
½ medium red onion, diced
2 T. honey or apple juice concentrate
½ cup carrot or zucchini, shredded
½ cup fresh tomatoes, chopped
1 ½ cups Italian-style tomato sauce (natural, low-sodium variety)
1 t. dried basil
1 t. dried oregano
1 15-oz. can black beans, rinsed and mashed or left whole (according to your preference)

Place garlic, onion, juice concentrate, carrot, and tomatoes in large skillet and cook over medium-high heat for 3 minutes. Add Italian-style tomato sauce, spices, and black beans and bring to a boil. Reduce heat to medium and continue to cook for about 10 to 15 minutes until it thickens.

Optional: For a heartier sauce, add ½ lb. crumbled cooked ground turkey breast or veggie burger.

African Coconut Peanut Tofu (serves 3–4)

2 cloves fresh garlic, minced
½ cup fat-free chicken or veggie broth
½ large onion, chopped
½ large carrot, chopped
1 stalk celery, chopped
½ large red bell pepper, chopped
1 lb. firm-style tofu, cut into large cubes
Sauce:
½ cup water or broth
2 T. wheat-free tamari or low-sodium soy sauce
3 cloves garlic, chopped
1 t. turmeric
½ t. ground ginger (or 2 tsp. fresh, chopped ginger)
⅛ t. cayenne pepper (use more to taste)
4 T. natural peanut butter

2 T. unsweetened coconut, flake or shredded
1 medium fresh orange (juice only)
Toppings: chopped peanuts, raisins/currants, yogurt (optional)

Stir-fry first six ingredients (not tofu) in large saucepan for 5 minutes or until veggies are slightly tender (add more broth if pan is too dry). Add tofu cubes and cook for 2 more minutes (stir gently so as not to break up tofu).

In another small saucepan, add all sauce ingredients and cook over medium-low heat until sauce is smooth and starts to thicken. Note: This sauce can be made ahead and stored in refrigerator. Reheat before serving, may need to add water.

Add sauce to the cooked veggies/tofu, and toss until well coated. Serve over Ginger Sesame Noodles *(follows)*. Add optional toppings on the side for an extra touch.

Ginger Sesame Rice Noodles (serves 4)
Sauce:
2 T. fresh orange juice
2 T. rice or white wine vinegar
2 cloves fresh garlic, minced or crushed
2 T. wheat-free tamari or low-sodium soy sauce
2 t. sesame oil (optional)
1 T. toasted sesame seeds
2 cups rice noodles or any style wheat-free noodles you like, cooked according to package directions
½ cup chopped scallions/green onions
¼ cup chopped cilantro
1 T. toasted sesame seeds (save for topping)

Mix sauce (first six ingredients) together in bowl; set aside.

In large saucepan, add sauce, cooked noodles, and green onion, and cook over medium heat until hot throughout (about 2 to 3 minutes). Toss hot noodles with cilantro and remaining seeds and serve.

Serving ideas: Add tofu or veggie burger for a main dish, or serve as side dish.

Nancy's Un-Meatballs and Un-Meatloaf (serves 12)
2 cups mixed (unsalted) raw nuts (almonds, pecans, etc.)
2 cups oat bran
1 cup oatmeal
1 cup chpped red onion
4 cloves garlic, minced
½ cup apple juice
4 T. wheat-free tamari or low-sodium soy sauce
1 cup low-fat ricotta cheese
½ cup grated low-fat mozzarella cheese
4 T. chopped parsley
2 t. sage
1 t. onion powder
2 t. thyme
1 t. ginger
¼ t. cayenne pepper (to taste)

Preheat oven to 350 degrees.

Blend nuts in food processor until finely ground.

In large bowl, mix oat bran, oatmeal, and ground nuts; add all the spices and chopped parsley and set aside. In iron skillet pan over medium heat, cook onion and garlic in apple juice and tamari until onions are clear.

Add onions to dry mixture and return to food processor; blend until smooth. Add ricotta cheese and mozzarella cheese and continue to blend until well mixed (add some water if too dry to blend). Return to bowl and add enough additional water until the mixture is at a consistency that can be made into meatballs and will hold together well (like meatloaf dough). Dip hands into a clean bowl of water and place 1 T. of mixture into wet hand and roll into balls. Place meatballs onto cookie sheet sprayed with nonstick spray.

Bake for 20–30 minutes until crispy brown on outside. Serve over wheat-free pasta and a natural spaghetti sauce or as appetizers with the spaghetti sauce for dipping.

For meatloaf: Place into small bread pans. Baking time will increase 15–20 minutes.

Sesame Tamari Tangerine Woking Chicken with Crunchy Veggies and 7-Grain Pilaf (serves 6–8)

4 medium boneless, skinless chicken breasts, cut into cubes

4 cloves fresh garlic, sliced thin or minced

¼ cup ginger tamari sauce *(recipe follows)*

2 t. toasted sesame oil (optional)

½ cup chopped scallions

1 cup chopped red cabbage

1 chopped large yellow or red bell pepper

½ cup ginger tamari sauce *(follows)*

or

½ cup chicken broth or water

2 cups cooked 7-grain mix (Kashi) or brown rice

2 small tangerines, peeled, separated, and cut into pieces

or

2 small cans (no sugar added) mandarin oranges, drained

¼ cup toasted sesame seeds

¼ cup chopped cilantro

Cook 7-grain mix or brown rice according to package directions. This can be done ahead of time.

In wok, iron skillet, or a nonstick pan, place garlic, ¼ cup Ginger Tamari Sauce, sesame oil, scallions, and chicken; cook over medium-high heat until the meat is white throughout. Add cabbage, bell pepper, ½ cup Ginger Tamari Sauce or broth, and cooked 7-grains, and continue to cook until veggies are desired texture. Add more broth or water if too dry. Stir in remaining ingredients and cook for 3 to 5 minutes or until heated throughout.

Ginger Tamari Sauce

1 cup wheat-free tamari or low-sodium tamari sauce

½ cup honey or apple juice concentrate

2 T. finely minced fresh ginger, or 2 t. ground ginger

Add any seasonings that you desire (pepper, herbs, etc.)

In iron skillet, bring all ingredients to a boil. Cook over medium heat for two minutes or until mixture starts to thicken. Remove from heat and let cool.

The sauce may be used to marinate the food that will be used in the shish-kebobs or for stir-fry (example: tofu, chicken, veggies). Pour sauce over food and place in covered container in the refrigerator overnight, or add to hot skillet for stir-fry.

This sauce can be made ahead of time and stored in covered container in refrigerator.

Lentil, Brown Rice, and Adzuki Bean Chili (serves 4–6)

3 15-oz. cans fat-free chicken or veggie broth
2 cups water or carrot juice (for a richer flavor)
1 cup brown rice (uncooked)
1 ½ cup lentils (if available, red lentils are more colorful)
1 large onion, chopped
3 cloves fresh garlic, minced
3 large carrots, chopped
1 large stalk celery, chopped
1 ½ T. chili powder
1 t. dried basil
1 t. dried oregano
1 t. dried thyme
1 15-oz. can whole tomatoes with juice
1 15-oz. can adzuki beans or black beans, rinsed and drained
1 cup Italian-style spaghetti sauce (fat-free variety)
½ cup chopped scallions (optional)
½ cup fresh basil or cilantro (optional)
½ cup low-fat grated cheddar or parmesan cheese (optional)

In large, heavy saucepan, add first 11 ingredients and bring to a boil. Reduce to simmer, cover pan, and allow to cook approximately 40 minutes or until rice and lentils are tender (may need to stir occasionally and add more water if too thick). Remove from heat and add tomatoes, adzuki beans, and Italian sauce. Return to heat and cook for about 10 more minutes. Top with optional toppings. Serve with crusty wheat-free bread or with warmed corn tortillas. Stores great for 2 weeks in the refrigerator!

Chunky Harvest Vegetable, Bean, and Barley Stew (serves 8–12)

2 T. white wine or chicken or veggie broth
4 T. wheat-free tamari or low-sodium soy sauce
1 large onion, finely chopped
3 cloves garlic, sliced
1 lb. fresh mushrooms, sliced
2 15-oz. cans fat-free chicken or veggie broth

2 cups water (or more broth for a richer flavor)
1 cup pearl barley, uncooked
1 t. thyme leaves, crushed
1 t. tarragon leaves, crushed
2 medium carrots, chopped
1 15-oz. can white beans, rinsed and drained
1 cup fresh-off-the-cob or frozen corn
1 cup frozen green peas
1 cup red pepper, chopped
2 cups shredded cooked chicken breast (optional)
1 ½ cups firm-style tofu, cubed (optional)

In large pan, sauté the first 5 ingredients until tender. Add the remaining ingredients and bring to a boil. Reduce the heat and simmer for about 45 minutes or until barley is tender. Serve with optional toppings (shredded chicken or tofu).

South-of-the-Border Corn, Bean, and Squash Stew (serves 8–12)
1 cup mild salsa (low-sodium variety)
2 cloves garlic, sliced
1 medium onion, finely chopped
2 medium zucchini or yellow summer squash, diced
2 15-oz. cans fat-free chicken or veggie broth
1 ½ cups frozen or fresh-off-the-cob corn
2 15-oz. cans pinto or black beans (or one of each)
3 T. canned green chilies (mild)
2 t. ground cumin
1 can evaporated skim milk or soy milk
½ cup low-fat jack or pepper jack cheese, grated
Optional toppings & additions:
½ cup fresh cilantro, chopped
½ cup fresh tomatoes, diced
½ cup natural-brand light sour cream
½ cup natural-brand guacamole

In large pan sauté the first 4 ingredients for 5 minutes. Stir in the next 5 ingredients and bring stew to a boil. Reduce heat and allow to simmer for 5 more minutes. Remove from heat and stir in the evaporated milk. Return to heat and warm over medium-low heat until hot throughout (be careful not to burn or curdle). Stir in grated cheese and serve with optional toppings.

Creamy Broccoli & Almond Butter Soup (serves 6–8)
2 15-oz. cans fat-free chicken or veggie broth
1 cup water
1 cup white potato, diced into small pieces
½ cup chopped green onion
2 cloves fresh garlic, minced
1 large carrot, chopped
2 cups chopped broccoli (reserve ½ cup of florets)
½ cup almond butter (or peanut butter)
2 t. no-salt seasoning blend (all-purpose blend)
Optional toppings:
¼ cup toasted chopped or sliced almonds
½ cup cilantro, chopped
½ cup carrot, grated

In large saucepan, add first 7 ingredients (do not use ½ cup of broccoli florets) and bring to a boil. Reduce heat to simmer, cover, and cook for 15 minutes or until veggies are tender. *Optional*: Blend in food processor for creamy-style.

Remove from the heat and stir in almond butter, seasonings, and reserved ½ cup broccoli florets until completely blended throughout. Return to low heat and allow to simmer for about 3–5 minutes (do not allow to boil).

Serve with optional toppings. Great with crusty bread or with warmed corn tortillas. Stores great for up to 2 weeks in the refrigerator.

Nancy's Crunchy and Colorful Chinese Coleslaw (serves 8–12)
4 cups chopped or granted red cabbage
1 large carrot, grated
½ cup chopped green or red bell pepper
½ cup chopped green onions
4 T. sliced almonds, toasted*
4 T. sunflower seeds, toasted*
2 T. sesame seeds, toasted*
1 package rice noodles
4 T. rice or balsamic vinegar
½ cup non-fat vanilla or plain yogurt
2 T. honey or fruit juice concentrate
2 cloves fresh garlic, minced
1 pkg. flavor packet from rice noodles

*To toast nuts/seeds, place in nonstick pan on medium heat and cook for 1–2 minutes until lightly browned. Remove from pan immediately. Be careful not to burn. Break noodles up into small pieces and cook noodles per instructions on the package; do not add flavor packet. When noodles are done, drain and set aside. Place first 7 ingredients in a large bowl and add noodles. In a small jar with a lid or a small mixing bowl, mix yogurt, vinegar, honey, and flavor packet. Whisk to create dressing. (This is a great dressing for any salad.) Add dressing to noodle/vegetable mixture and chill to serve.

Serving ideas: Add chicken, seafood, or tofu for an excellent main-dish salad for lunch or a light dinner, or stuff in a corn tortilla. Excellent source of beta carotene & vitamin C.

Nancy's High-Energy Multi-Bean and Rice Bake (serves 8–12)
2 cups brown rice (regular or quick cooking)
3 15-oz. cans beans (black, kidney, garbanzo, etc.)
½ cup fresh or natural-brand salsa (chunky style)
1 clove garlic, minced
½ large red onion, chopped
2 t. cumin
2 cups natural-brand spaghetti sauce (low-fat and low-sodium style)
10 dashes Tabasco sauce
1 cup fat-free cheddar cheese
½ cup parmesan cheese

Preheat oven to 350 degrees. Cook rice according to package directions and set aside. Rinse canned beans thoroughly in a colander.

In a large glass baking dish, combine salsa, garlic, onions, and cumin. Cook in microwave on high for 2 minutes until onions are soft (or cook on stove in a nonstick skillet). Add beans, tomato sauce, and Tabasco; stir together until mixed.

Place cooked rice in the bottom of a 13 x 9 baking pan, cover with bean mixture, and top with grated cheeses. Place in oven and bake 15–20 minutes until hot throughout.

For a quicker method, microwave the casserole for approximately 5 minutes on high.

Spicy Black Bean and Corn Chili (serves 10–12)
1 medium red onion, chopped
¼ cup chicken broth or apple juice
3 cloves garlic, chopped
1 cup zucchini, chopped
1 cup green bell pepper, chopped
2 cups frozen or fresh-off-the-cob corn
2 15-oz. cans whole tomatoes
½ cup natural-brand chunky-style salsa
2 15-oz. cans black beans
2 T. chili powder
1 t. cumin
1 t. oregano

Rinse beans in colander to remove excess salt.

In a large saucepan or skillet, sauté the first 5 ingredients over medium-high heat for 2 minutes or until vegetables are softened. Add the remaining ingredients to the pan and bring to a boil. Reduce heat to simmer and continue to cook for 20 minutes, covered, stirring occasionally.

Optional ingredients: Include one of the following ingredients and allow to cook until meat is completely cooked: tofu, chicken breast, or ground turkey breast.

To-Die-For Creamy Carrot Spiced Shakes (serves 2)
1 cup carrot juice (fresh or bottled)
½ medium frozen banana*
1 cup vanilla non-fat frozen yogurt (or ice milk)
1 T. raisins
1 T. chopped dates
1 t. cinnamon (or less to taste)
1 T. sliced raw almonds

*Peel very ripe banana and wrap in wax paper and freeze.

Slice the frozen banana into small pieces. Place all the ingredients into blender, and blend until smooth.

Variations: Use any combination of fresh or frozen fruits, juices, and dried fruits. This is a very energizing and flavorful drink!

Appendix Section 6

Yeast-free diet

Candida albicans is dependent on simple carbohydrates for growth. You must strictly avoid yeast-containing foods in order to be successful on this diet. The following are guidelines for you to follow.

Sugars
Do not eat sugars or sweets. This includes all products made with honey, molasses, sucrose, or syrup.

Grains
You may eat the following whole grains:
Millet, buckwheat, amaranth, rice, corn, quinoa, oats. Attempt to use a wide variety of these grains in order to avoid using high-gluten-containing grains. Grains with a high gluten content (wheat, rye, and barley) should be restricted.

Avoid all enriched grains. This means avoid all grains that have been fortified with synthetic nutrients or additives during processing.

Dairy products
You may eat the following dairy products:
Butter, cream, sour cream, cream cheese, Neufchatel cheese, cottage cheese, kefir cheese, plain kefir, plain yogurt, and buttermilk.

Avoid all forms of brick cheese, blue cheese, camembert, etc.
Avoid milk.

Fruit

You may eat up to two pieces of fruit per day. However, fruit juices must be temporarily omitted from the diet. Berries, apples, pears, avocados, and tomatoes are acceptable. Freshness reduces mold buildup.

Avoid citrus fruits and fruits that have high mold content. Melons, especially cantaloupe and the skins of fleshy fruits such as peaches and apricots, fall into this category. Avoid dried fruits such as prunes, raisins, dates, figs, candied cherries, and currants. Avoid canned or frozen fruits including those containing citric acid.

Nuts

You may eat fresh whole nuts and seeds, including their butters and milks. Avoid peanuts and pistachios and dry-roasted nuts.

Vegetables

Vegetables are highly encouraged on this diet. You may eat them raw or cooked. Fresh tofu is also acceptable. Avoid mushrooms.

Legumes

You may eat legumes and their sprouts if very fresh. Legumes are beans, peas, peapods, soybeans, lentils, etc. They can be cooked for soups and stews or cold for salads.

Yeast

Yeast is used in food preparation and handling so be sure to avoid all commercial breads, rolls, coffee cakes, pastries, etc. Beer, wine, and all alcoholic beverages should be avoided. Vinegar and vinegar-containing foods such as pickled vegetables, sauerkraut, relish, green olives, and salad dressing should also be avoided. Lemon or lime juice with oil may be used as a salad dressing. Soy sauce, cider, and natural root beer; most commercial soups and barbecue chips; pickled, smoked or dried meats; fish and poultry, including sausages, salami, tongue, corned beef, pastrami, bacon, and any type of country-style cured pork should all be avoided. Avoid any vitamins or mineral supplements that contain yeast.

Miscellaneous

Dried herb teas and spices are acceptable. Coffee beans are fermented and dried and should be avoided. Coffee and black teas should be avoided due to caffeine content.

What is left to eat?
Proteins: Fish, chicken, beef, pork, turkey, duck, seafood of all kinds, eggs, goat, venison, rabbit, frog legs, pheasant, quail, lamb, and veal.
Vegetables, legumes, grains, and fruits as noted above.

Is it possible to eat out?
Yes! Just order carefully and skip the cocktail. Have oil and lemon juice on your salad. Order chicken, fish, or other animal protein that is prepared without sauces. Broiled or plain items are the safest. Steamed vegetables are perfect. Skip bread, crackers, and dessert.

If you are aware of specific allergies to any of the allowed foods, you must avoid those foods also. Contact us if you have any questions.

Alternative Foods for a Yeast-free Diet

Flours
Amaranth
Arrowroot
Artichoke (Jerusalem)
Buckwheat
Cassava
Chickpea
Lima Bean
Lotus Root
Malanga
Nut and Seed Flours
Oat
Potato
Quinoa
Rice
Sesame
Soybean
Tapioca
Water Chestnut
Sweet Potato
Yam

Leavenings
Baking Soda
Baking Powder
Featherweight Baking Powder

Thickeners
Arrowroot Starch
Agar Agar
Buckwheat Flakes
Malanga Starch
Potato Starch
Rice Starch
Tapioca Starch

Milk Substitute
Vegetable Juices

Zucchini Milk
Goat Milk
Nut or Seed Milk, "Energy Quick"
by Energy Foods
Almond Meal
Potato Milk
Soy Milk
Milk: Special Foods (Cassava, Lotus
Root, Malanga, Water Chestnut,
White Sweet Potato)

Cereals and Meals
Amaranth (puffed and cereal)
Buckwheat (cereal and flakes)
Creamed Cereals: Special Foods
(Lotus Root, Amaranth, etc.)
Crispy Cereal Shreds: Special Foods
(Malanga, Cassava, Yam, etc.)
Millet Flakes
Rice (cereal and puffed)
Quinoa (puffed and cereal)

Pastas and Noodles
Bifun (rice and potato)
Buckwheat
Green Bean Noodles
Kuzi Kuri
Mung Bean Noodles
Pasta: Special Foods (Amaranth,
Cassava, Yam, Etc.)
Saifun (sweet potato starch)

Vegetable Chips
Artichoke Chips
Carrot Chips
Cassava Chips
Malanga Chips
Parsnip Chips

Potato Chips
Rice Petals
Sweet Potato Chips

Oils
Almond
Apricot Kernel
Avocado
Beef Drippings
Canola Oil
Chicken Fat
Coconut
Cottonseed
Olive
Palm Kernel
Pumpkin
Safflower
Sesame
Soy
Sunflower

Egg Alternatives
Arrowroot Mixture
Baking Powder Mixture
Egg Replacer
Flaxseed Mixture
Soybean Curd

Crackers
Amaranth
Cassava
Brown Rice
Lotus Root
Malanga
White Sweet Potato
Yam

Resources

American Academy of Environmental Medicine
6505 E. Central Ave. #296
Wichita, KS 67206
Phone: 316-684-5500
Fax: 316-684-5709
Email: adminstrator@aaemonline.org

American College for Advancement in Medicine
8001 Irvine Center Dr. #825
Irvine, CA 92618
Phone: 800-532-3668
                949-309-3520
Fax: 949-309-3538
Website: www.acam.org

American Academy of Anti-Aging Medicine
1510 W. Montana St.
Chicago, IL 60614
Phone: 773-528-1000
Fax: 773-528-5390
Email: info@worldhealth.net

American Holistic Medical Association
23366 Commerce Park #101B
Beachwood, OH 44122
Phone: 216-292-6644
Fax: 216-292-6688
Email: info@holisticmedicine.org

The Institute for Functional Medicine
4411 Pt. Fosdick Dr. NW #305
P.O. box 1697
Gig Harbor, WA 98335
Phone: 800-228-0622
                253-858-4724
Fax: 253-853-6766
Email: client_services@fxmed.com

References

Abidov, M., Grachev, S., Seifulla, R.D., Ziegenfuss, T.N. Extract of Rhodiola rosea radix reduces the level of C-reactive protein and creatinine kinase in the blood. *Bull Exp Biol Med.* Jul 2004;138(1):63-4.

al'Absi, M., Lovallo, W.R., McKey, B., Sung, B.H., Whitsett, T.L., Wilson, M.F. Hypothalamic-pituitary-adrenocortical responses to psychological stress and caffeine in men at high and low risk for hypertension. *Psychosom Med.* Jul-Aug 1998;60(4):521-7.

Abbey, M., Noakes, M., Belling, G.B., Nestel, P.J. Partial replacement of saturated fatty acids with almonds or walnuts lowers total plasma cholesterol and low-density-lipoprotein cholesterol. *Am J Clin Nutr.* 1997;59:995-9.

Adlercreutz, C.H., Golden, B.R., Gorbach, S.L., Soybean phytoestrogen intake and cancer risk. *J Nutr.* Mar 1995;125 Suppl 3:S757-70.

Agerholm-Larsen, L., Raben, A., Haulrik, N., Effect of 8-week intake of probiotic milk products on risk factors for cardiovascular diseases. *Eur J Clin Nutr.* Apr 2000;54(4):288-97.

Aggarwal, B.B., Kumar, A., Bharti, A.C. Anticancer potential of curcumin: preclinical and clinical studies. *Anticancer Res.* Jan 2003;23(1A):363-98.

Ahonen, M.H., Tenkanen, L., Teppo, L., Hakama, M., Tuohimaa, P. Prostate cancer risk and prediagnostic serum 25-hydroxyvitamin D levels (Finland). *Cancer Causes Control.* 2000;11:847-52.

Alele, J.D., Kamen, D.L. The importance of inflammation and vitamin D status in SLE-associated osteoporosis. *Autoimmun Rev.* May 7 2009. Epub ahead of print.

Allgood, V.E., Powell-Oliver, F.E., Cidlowski, J.A. Vitamin B6 influences glucocorticoid receptor-dependent gene expression. *J Biol Chem.* 1990;265:12324-433.

Allgood, V.E., Powell-Oliver, F.E., Cidlowski, J.A. The influence of vitamin B6 on the structure and function of the glucocorticoid receptor. *Ann N Y Acad Sci.* 1990;585:452-65.

Anagnostis, P., Athyros, V.G., The pathogenetic role of cortisol in the metabolic syndrome: a hypothesis. *J Clin Endocrinol Metab.* May 26 2009;94(8):2692-701.

Anderson, D.A., Shapiro, J.R., Lundgren, J.D., Spataro, L.E., Frye, C.A. Self-reported dietary restraint is associated with elevated levels of salivary cortisol. *Appetite.* Feb 2002;38(1):13-7.

Anderson, J.W., Deakins, D.A., Floore, T.L., Smith, B.M., Shitis, S.E. Dietary fiber and coronary heart disease. *Crit Rev Food Sci Nutr.* 1990;29(2):95-147.

Anderson, J.W., Gustafson, N.J., Spencer, D.B., Tietyen J., Bryant, C.A. Serum lipid response of hypercholesterolemic men to single and divided doses of canned beans. *Am J Clin Nutr.* Jun 1990;51(6):1013-9.

Anderson, J.W., Johnstone, B.M., Cook-Newell, M.E. Meta-analysis of the effects of soy protein intake on serum lipids. *N Engl J Med.* Aug 3 1995;333(5):276-82.

Anderson, J.W., Gustafson, N.J. Hypocholesterolemic effects of oat and bean products. *Am J Clin Nutr.* Sep 1988;48 Suppl 3:S749-53.

Andrew, R., Gale, C., Walker, B., Seckl, J., Martyn, C.N. Glucocorticoid metabolism and the metabolic syndrome: associations in an elderly cohort. *Exp Clin Endocrinol Diabetes.* Sep 2002;110(6):284-90.

Andrews, R.C., Herlihy, O., Livingston, D.E., Andrew, R., Walker, B.R. Abnormal cortisol metabolism and tissue sensitivity to cortisol in patients with glucose intolerance. *J Clin Endocrinol Metab.* Dec 2002;87(12):5587-93.

Apstolova, G., Schweizer, R.A., Balazs, Z., Kostadinova, R.M., Odermatt, A. Dehydroepiandrosterone inhibits the amplification of glucocorticoid action in adipose tissue. *Am J Physiol Endocrinol Metab.* May 2005;288(5):E957-64.

Askari, H., Liu, J., Dagogo, J.S. Energy adaptation to glucocorticoid-induced hyperleptinemia in human beings. *Metabolism.* Jul 2005;54(7):876-80.

Atanasov, A.G., Dzyakanchuk, A.A., Schweizer, R.A., Nashev, L.G., Maurer, E.M., Odermatt, A. Coffee inhibits the reactivation of glucocorticoids by 11beta-hydroxysteroid dehydrogenase type 1: a glucocorticoid connection in the anti-diabetic action of coffee? *FEBS Lett.* Jul 2006;580(17):4081-5.

Aybak, M., Sermet, A., Ayyildiz, M.O., Karakilcik, A.Z. Effect of oral pyridoxine hydrocholoride supplementation on arterial blood pressure in patients with essential hypertension. *Arzneimittelforschung.* 1995;45:1271-3.

Babio, N. Bullo, M. Salas-Salvado,J. Mediterranean diet and metabolic syndrome:the evidence. *Public Health Nutr.* Sep 2009;12(9A):1607-17.

Bahr, V., Pfeiffer, A.F., Diederich, S. The metabolic syndrome X and peripheral cortisol synthesis. *Exp Clin Endocrinol Diabetes.* Oct 2002;110(7):313-8.

Balbio N, Bullo M et al Adherence to the Mediterranean diet and risk of metabolic syndrome, *Nutr Metab Cardiovasc Dis.* Oct 2009;19(8): 563-70

Baldewicz, T., Goodkin, K., Feaster, D.J., Blaney, N.T., Kumar, M., Kuman, A., et al. Plasma pyridoxine deficiency is related to increased psychological distress in recently bereaved homosexual men. *Psychosom Med.* 1998;60:297-308.

Basu, R., Breda, E., Aberg, A.L., Mechanisms of the age-associated deterioration in glucose tolerance: contribution of alterations in insulin secretion, action, and clearance. *Diabetes.* 2003;52:1738-48.

Bauer, M.E. Stress, glucocorticoids and ageing of the immune system. *Stress.* Mar 2005;8(1):69-83.

Beckman, K.B., Ames, B.N. The free radical theory of aging matures. *Physiol Rev.* 1998;78:547-81.

Behrens, S., Ehlers, C., Bruggemann, T., Ziss, W., Dissman, R., Galecka, M., et al. Modification of the circadian pattern of ventricular tachyarrhythmias by beta-blocker therapy. *Clin Cardiol.* 1997;20:247-253.

Belch, J.J., Ansell, D., Madhok, R. Effects of altering dietary essential fatty acids on requirements for non-steroidal anti-inflammatory drugs in patient with rheumatoid arthritis: a double blind placebo controlled study. *Ann Rheum Dis.* 1988;47(2):96-104.

Belch, J.J., Hill, A. Evening primrose oil and borage oil in rheumatologic conditions. *Am J Clin Nutri.* 2000;71 Suppl:S352-6.

Bhathena, S.J., Velasquez, M.T. Beneficial role of dietary phytoestrogens in obesity and diabetes. *Am J Clin Nutr.* Dec 2002;76(6):1191-201.

Bhattacharya, S. Anti-stress activity of sitoindosides VII and VIII, new acylsterylglucosides from Withania somnifera. *Phytother Res.* 1987;1:32-7.

Bjorntorp, P., Rosmond, R. The metabolic syndrome: a neuroendocrine disorder? *Br J Nutr.* 2000;83 Suppl 1:S49-57.

Bjorntorp, P. Do stress reactions cause abdominal obesity and comorbidities? *Obes Rev.* May 2001;2(2):73-86.

Bjorntorp, P. Stress and cardiovascular disease. *Icta Physiol Scand Suppl.* 1997;640:144-8.

Bjorntorp, P. Visceral fat accumulation: the missing link between psychosocial factors and cardiovascular disease? *J Intern Med.* 1991;230:195-201.

Bjorntorp, P., Holm, G., Rosmond, R. Hypothalamic arousal, insulin resistance and type 2 diabetes mellitus. *Diabetes Med.* 1999;16:373-383.

Black, P.H. The inflammatory consequences of psychologic stress: relationship to insulin resistance, obesity, atherosclerosis and diabetes mellitus, type II. *Med Hypotheses.* 2006;67(4):879-91.

Bland, J.S., Bralley, J.A. Nutritional regulation of hepatic detoxification enzymes. *J Appl Nutr.* 1991;44(3&4):2-15.

Bloedon, L.T., Szapary, P.O. Flaxseed and cardiovascular risk. *Nutr Rev.* Jan 2004;62(1):18-27.

Bomba, A., Nemcova, R., Gancarcikova, E. The influence of omega-3 polyunsaturated fatty acids (omega-3 pufa) on lactobacilli adhesion to the intestinal mucosa and on immunity in gnotobiotic piglets. *Berl Munch Tierarztl Wochenschr.* Jul 2003;116(7-8):312-6.

Borchers, A.T., Kean, C.L., Gershwin, M.E. The influence of yogurt/ Lactobacillus on the innate and acquired immune response. *Clin Rev Allergy Immunol.* Jun 2002:22(3):207-30.

Borkman, M., Campbell, L.V., Chisholm, D.J., Storlien, L.H. Comparison of the effects on insulin sensitivity of high carbohydrate and high fat diets in normal subjects. *J Clin Endocrinol Metab.* 1991;72:432-7.

Braly, J. Holford, P. Hidden food allergies. Laguna Beach: Basic Health Publications; 2006.

Brand-Miller, J.C., et al. Glycemic index and obesity. *Am J Clin Nutr.* 2002;76(1):281S-5S.

Brenneman, J.C. Allergy elimination diet as the most effective gallbladder diet. *Ann Allergy.* 1968;26:83-7.

Brouet, I., Ohshima, H. Curcumin, an anti-tumour promoter and anti-inflammatory agent, inhibits induction of nitric oxide synthase in activated macrophages. *Biochem Biophys Res Commun.* Jan 17 1995;206(2):533-40.

Brown, D., Gaby, A., Reichert, R. Phytotherapeutic and nutritional approaches to diabetes mellitus. *Quarterly Rev Nat Med.* 1998;Winter:329-51.

Bruder, E.D., Raff, H., Goodfriend, T.L. An oxidized derivative of linoleic acid stimulates dehydroepiandrosterone production by human adrenal cells. *Horm Metab Res.* Dec 2006;38(12):803-6.

Brunner, E., Hemingway, H., Walker, B., Page M., Clarke P., Juneja, M. Adrenocortical, autonomic, and inflammatory causes of the nested case-control study. *Circulation.* Nov 19 2002;106(21):2659-65.

Bujalska, I.J., Kumar, S., Stewart, P.M. Does central obesity reflect Cushing's disease of the omentum? *Lancet.* 1997;349:1210-3.

Burgess, J.R., Stevens, L., Zhang, W., Peck, L. Long-chain polyunsaturated fatty acids in children with attention-deficit hyperactive disorder. *Am J Clin Nutri.* 2000;71 Suppl:S327-30.

Bustamante, J., Lodge, J.K., Marcocci, L. Alpha-lipoic acid in liver metabolism and disease. *Free Rad Biol Med.* 1998;24(6):1023-39.

Buydens-Branchey, L. Low HDL cholesterol, aggression and altered central serotonergic activity. *Psychiatry Res.* Mar 6 2000;93(2):93-102.

Calorie Restriction Society Web site. http://www.calorierestriction.org/. Accessibility verified February 5, 2007.

Carr, D.J., Guarcello, V., Blalock, J.E. Phosphatidylserine suppresses antigen-specific IgM production by mice orally administered sheep red blood cells. *Proc Soc Exp Biol Med.* Sep 1992;200(4):548-54.

Carroll, D.N., Roth, M.T. Evidence for the cardioprotective effects of omega-3 fatty acids. *Ann Pharmacother.* 2002;36(12):1950-6.

Celiac Disease Statistics, Jefferson University Hospitals Division of gastroenterology and hepatology. *NIH Publication No. 98-4269* April 1998.

Chainani-Wu, N. Safety and anti-inflammatory activity of curcumin: a component of turmeric (Curcuma longa). *J Altern Complement Med.* Feb 2003;9(1):161-8.

Charmandari, E., Weise, M., Bornstein, S., Eisenhofer, G., Keil, M. Children with classic congenital adrenal hyperplasia have elevated serum leptin concentrations and insulin resistance: potential clinical implications. *J Clin Endocrinol Metab.* May 2002;87(5):2114-20.

Chee, K.M., Gong, J.X., Rees, D.M.G., Meydani, M., Ausman, L., Johnson, J., et al. Fatty acid content of marine oil capsules. *Lipids* 25, 1990:523-527.

Chen, J., Stavro, P.M., Thompson, L.U. Dietary flaxseed inhibits human breast cancer growth and metastasis and downregulates expression of insulin-like growth factor and epidermal growth factor receptor. *Nutr Cancer.* 2002;43(2):187-92.

Christiansen, E., Schnider, S., Palmvig, B., Tauber-Lassen, E., Pedersen, O. Intake of a diet high in trans monounsaturated fatty acids or saturated fatty acids: effects on postprandial insulinemia and glycemia in obese patients with NIDDM. *Diabetes Care.* 1997;20:881-7.

Coiro, V., Casti, A., Rubino, P., Manfredi, G., Maffei, M.L., Melani, A., et al. Free fatty acids inhibit adrenocorticotropin and cortisol secretion stimulated by physical exercise in normal men. *Clin Endocrinol (Oxf).* May 2007;66(5):740-3.

Coles, L.S. Table of world-wide living supercentenarians. *J Anti Aging Med.* 2002;5:231-3.

Compton, M.M., Cidlowski, J.A. Vitamin B6 and glucocorticoid action. *Endocr Rev.* 1986;7:140-8.

Connor, W.E. Importance of n-3 fatty acids in health and disease. *Am J Clin Nutr.* 2000;71 Suppl:S171-5.

Corral, A.R., Sierra-Johnson, J., Orban, M., Gami, A.S., Kuniyoshi, R.H.S., Pusalavidyasager, S., et al. Modest fat gain causes endothelial dysfunction in lean healthy humans: a randomized blinded controlled trial. *Circulation.* 2007;116:16 Suppl:797.

Costa R.J., Jones G.E. The effects of a high carbohydrate diet on cortisol and salivary immunoglobulin A (s-IgA) during a period of increase exercise workload amongst Olympic and Ironman triathletes. *Int J Sports Med.* Dec 2005;26(10):880-5.

Cynober, L.A. Plasma amino acid levels with a note on membrane transport: characteristics, regulation, and metabolic significance. *Nutrition.* Sep 2002;18(9):761-6.

D'Souza, A.L., Raijkumar, C., Cooke, J., Bulpitt, C.J. Probiotics in prevention of antibiotic associated diarrhoea: meta-analysis. *BMJ.* Jun 8 2002;324(7350):1361.

Dakshinamurti, K., Sharma, S.K., Bonke, D. Influence of B vitamins on binding properties of serotonin receptors in the CNS of rats. *Klin Wochenschr.* 1990;688:142-5.

Dakshinamurti, K., Paulose, C.S., Viswanathan, M., Siow, Y.L. Neuroendocrinology of pyridoxine deficiency. *Neurosci Biobehav Rev.* 1988;12:189-93.

Danescu, L.G., Levy, S. Vitamin D and diabetes mellitus. *Endocrine.* Feb 2009;35(1):11-7.

Delarue, J., Matzinger, O., Binnert, C., Schneiter, P., Chiolero, M.R., Tappy, L. Fish oil prevents the adrenal activation elicited by mental stress in healthy men. *Diabetes Metab.* Jun 2003;29(3):289-95.

de Prada, T.P., Pozzi, A.O. Atherogenesis takes place in cholesterol-fed rabbits when circulating concentrations of endogenous cortisol are increased and inflammation suppressed. *Atherosclerosis.* Jun 24 2006;191(2):235-470.

Dhabhar, F.S., Miller, A.H., McEwen, B.S., Spencer, R.L. Effects of stress on immune cell distribution: dynamics and hormonal mechanisms. *J Immunol.* 1995;154:5511-27.

Dhingra, R., Sullivan, L., Jacques, P.F., Wang, T.J., Fox, C.S., Meigs J.B., et al. Soft drink consumption and risk of developing cardiometabolic risk factors and the metabolic syndrome in middle-aged adults in the community. *Circulation.* Jul 31 2007;116(5):480-8.

Dixon, R.A. Phytoestrogens. *Annu Rev Plant Biol.* 2004;55:225-61.

Dyerbergt, J., Bang, H.O. Haemostatic function and platelet polyunsaturated fatty acids in Eskimos. *Lancet.* 1979;2(8140):433-5.

Egger,J., Will, J., Carter, CM. Is migraine food allergy? A double-blind control trial of oligoantigenic diet treatment *Lancet* 1983;865.

Eiji, T., Terao, J., Nakaya, Y., Miyamoto, K., Baba, Y., Chuman, H., et al. Stress control and human nutrition. *J. of Med Investigation.* Aug 4, 2004;51(3):139-145.

Faggiano, A., Pivonello, R., Melis, D., Alfieri, R., Filippela, M. Evaluation of circulating levels and renal clearance of natural amino acids in patients with Cushing's disease. *J Endocrinol Invest.* Feb 2002;25(2):142-51.

Fairfield, K.M., Fletcher, R.H. Vitamins for chronic disease prevention in adults: scientific review. *JAMA.* 2002;287:3116-26.

Fernandez-Real, J.M., Pugeat, M., Grasa, M., Broch, M., Vendrell, J., Brun, J., et al. Serum corticosteroid-binding globulin concentration and insulin resistance syndrome: a population study. *J Clin Endocrinol Metab.* Oct 2002;87(10):4686-90.

Feskens, E.J., Kromhout, D. Cardiovascular risk factors and the 25-year incidence of diabetes mellitus in middle-aged men: the Zutphen Study. *Am J Epidemio.* 1989;130:1101-8.

Folsom, A.R., Nieto, F.J., McGovern, P.G., Prospective study of coronary heart disease incidence in relation to fasting total homocysteine, related genetic polymorphisms, and B vitamins: the Atherosclerosis Risk in Communities (ARIC) study. *Circulation.* 1998;98:204-10.

Fontana, L., Meyer, T.E., Klein, S., Holloszy, J.O. Long-term calorie restriction is highly effective in reducing the risk for atherosclerosis in humans. *Proc Natl Acad Sci USA.* 2004;101:6659-63.

Fontana, L., Klein, S., Holloszy, J.O., Premachandra, B.N. Effect of long-term calorie restriction with adequate protein and micronutrients on thyroid hormones. *J Clin Endocrinol Metab.* 2006;91:3232-5.

Fortin, P.R., Lew, R.A., Liang, M.H. Validation of a meta-analysis: the effects of fish oil in rheumatoid arthritis. *J Clin Epidemiol.* 1995;48(11):1379-90.

Fries, E., Hesse, J., Hellhammer, J., Hellhammer, D.H. A new view on hypocortisolism. *Psychoneuroendocrinology.* Nov 2005:30 (10)1010-6.

Frisco, S, Low circulating vitamin B(6) is associated with elevation of the inflammation marker C-reactive protein independently of plasma homocysteine levels. *Circulation.* 2001;103:2788-91.

Fruehwald-Schultes, B., Kern, W., Born, J., Fehm, H.L., Peters, A. Hyperinsulinemia causes activation of the hypothalamus in humans. *Int J Obes Relat Metab Disord*. May 2001;25 Suppl 1:S38-40.

Gaffney, B.T., Hugel, H.M. The effects of Eleutherococcus senticosus and Panax ginseng on steroidal hormone indices of stress and lymphoctye subset numbers in endurance athletes. *Life Sci*. Dec 14 2001;70(4):431-42.

Garcia-Prieto, M.D., Tebar, F.J. Cortisol secretary pattern and glucocorticoid feedback sensitivity in women from a Mediterranean area: relationship with anthropometric characteristics, dietary intake and plasma fatty acid profile. *Clin Endocrinol (Oxf)*. Feb 2007;66(2):185-91.

Garland, C., Comstock, G., Garland, F. Serum 25-hydroxyvitamin D and colon cancer: eight year prospective study. *Lancet*. 1989;2:1176-8.

Gilbert, D.G., Dibb, W.D. Effects of nicotine and caffeine, separately and in combination, on EEG topography, mood, heart rate, cortisol, and vigilance. *Psychophysiology*. Sep 2000;37(5):583-95.

Gilchrest, B.A., Bohr, V.A. Aging processes, DNA damage, and repair. *FASEB J*. 1997;11:322-30.

Gluck, M.E., Geliebter, A., Lorence, M. Cortisol stress response is positively correlated with central obesity in obese women with binge eating disorder (BED) before and after cognitive-behavioral treatment. *Ann NY Acad Sci*. Dec 2004;1032:202-7.

Goldstein, D., McEwen, B.S. Allostasis, homeostasis, and the nature of stress. *Stress*. 2002;5:55-8.

Golub, M.D. The adrenal and the metabolic syndrome. *Curr Hypertens Rep*. 2001;3:117-20.

Gonzalez-Bono, E., Rohleder, N., Glucose but not protein or fat load amplifies the cortisol response to psychosocial stress. *Horm Behav*. May 2002;41(3):328-33.

Grant, E.C. Food allergies and migraine. *Lancet* May 5, 1979

Green, H.R., Jones, R. Celiac disease: a hidden epidemic. New York: Harper Collins; 2006.

Hamazaki, T., Itomura, M. Anti-stress effects of DHA. *Biofactors*. 2000;13(1-4):41-5.

Hamazaki, K., Itomura, M. Effect of omega-3 fatty acid-containing phospholipids on blood catecholamine concentrations in healthy volunteers: a randomized, placebo-controlled, double-blind trial. *Nutrition*. Jun 2005;21(6):705-10.

Han, E.S., Evans, T.R., Shu, J.H., Lee, S., Nelson, J.F. Food restriction enhances endogenous and corticotropin-induced plasma elevations of free but not total corticosterone throughout life in rats. *J Gerontol A Biol Sci Med Sci*. 2001;56:391-397.

Harris, W.S., Park, Y., Isley, W.L. Cardiovascular disease and long-chain omega-3 fatty acids. *Curr Opin Lipidol*. 2003;1q4(1):9-14.

Hartvig. P., Lindner, K.J., Bjurling, P., Laengsrom, B., Tedroff, J. Pyridoxine effect on synthesis rate of serotonin in the monkey brain measured with positron emission tomography. *J Neural Transm Gen Sect*. 1995;102:91-7.

Hartz, A.J., Bentler, S., Noyes, R., Hoehns, J., Logemann, C., Sinift, S. Randomized controlled trial of Siberian ginseng for chronic fatigue. *Psychol Med*. Jan 2004;34(1):51-61.

He K, Rimm, E.B., Merchant, A. Fish consumption and risk of stroke in men. *JAMA*. 2002;288(24):3130-6.

Heber, D. What does the adipocyte secrete? *PCRI Insights*. May 2004;7(4).

Heilbronn, L.K., de Jonge, L., Frisard, M.I. Effect of 6-month calorie restriction on biomarkers of longevity, metabolic adaptation, and oxidative stress in overweight individuals: a randomized controlled trail. *JAMA*. 2006;295:1539-48.

Hennig B., Reiterer, G., Modification of environmental toxicity by nutrients: implications in atherosclerosis. *Cardiovasc Toxicol*. 2005;5(2):153-60.

Herrick, K., Phillips, D.I., Haselden, S., Shiell, A.W., Campbell-Brown, M., Godfrey, K.M. Maternal consumption of a high-meat, low-carbohydrate diet in late pregnancy: relation to adult cortisol concentrations in the offspring. *J Clin Endocrinol Metab*. Aug 2003;88(8):3554-60.

Hjemdahl, P. Stress and the metabolic syndrome, an interesting but enigmatic association. *Circulation*. 2002;106:2634-6.

Hoffman, P.R., Kench, J.A., Vondracek, A. Interaction between phosphatidylserine and the phosphatidylserine receptor inhibits immune responses in vivo. *J Immunol*. Feb 2005;174(3):1393-404.

Hoj, L. A double-blind controlled trial of elemental diet in severe perennial asthma. *Allergy*. 1981;36(4):257-62.

Holick, M.F. High prevalence of vitamin D inadequacy and implications for health. *Mayo Clin Proc*. 2006;81:363-73.

Holloszy, J.L. The biology of aging. *Mayo Clin Proc*. 2000;75 Suppl:S3-8.

Horrobin, D.R. Fatty acid metabolism in health and disease: the role of delta-6-desaturase. *Am J Clin Nutr*. 1993;57 Suppl:S732-7.

Hougee, S., Sanders, A. Decreased pro-inflammatory cytokine production by LPS-stimulated PBMC upon in vitro incubation with the flavonoids, apigenin, luteolin or chrysin, due to selective elimination of monocytes/macrophases. *Biochem Pharmacol*. Jan 15 2005;69(2):241-8.

Hu, F.B., Stampfer, M.J., Manson, J.E. Dietary fat intake and the risk of coronary heart disease in women. *N Engl J Med*. 1997;337:1491-9.

Hypponen, E., Laara, E., Reunamen, A., Jarvelin, M.R., Virtanen, S.M. Intake of vitamin D and risk of type 1 diabetes: a birth cohort study. *Lancet*. 2001;358:1500-3.

Ika, T., Komori, N., Kuwahata, M., Hiroi, Y., Shimoda, T., Okada, M., et al. Pyridoxal 5-phosphate modulates expression of cytosolic aspartate aminotransferase gene by inactivation of glucocorticoid receptor. *J Nutr Sci Vitaminol (Tokyo)*. 1995;41:363-75.

Ishigaki, T., Koyama, K. Plasma leptin levels of elite endurance runners after heavy endurance training. *J Physiol Anthropol Appl Human Sci.* Nov 2005;24(6):573-8.

Jäger, R., Purpura, M., Geiss, K.R., Weib, M., Baumeister, J., Amatulli, F., et al. The effect of phosphatidylserine on golf performance. *J of the Intern Soc of Sports Nutrition.* Dec 2007;4:23.

James, M.J., Gibson, R.A., Cleland, L.G. Dietary polyunsaturated fatty acids and inflammatory mediator production. *Am J Clin Nutr.* 2000;71 Suppl:S343-8.

Janossky, E.D., Lester, G.E., Weinberg, C.R. Association between low levels of 1,25-dihydroxyvitamin D and breast cancer risk. *Public Health Nutr.* 1999;2:238-91.

Jayo, J.M., Shively, C.A., Kaplan, J.R., Manuck, S.B. Effects of exercise and stress on body fat distribution in male cynomolgus monkeys. *Int J Obes Relat Metab Disord.* 1993;17:597-604.

Jefferies, W.M. Cortisol and immunity. *Medical Hypotheses.* 1991;34:198-208.

Jeong, D.H., Lee, G.P . Alterations of mast cells and TGF-beta1 on the silymarin treatment for CCI(4)-induced hepatic fibrosis. *World J Gastroenterol.* Feb 28 2005;11(8):1141-8.

Jezova, D., Duncko, R., Lassanova, M., Kriska, M., Moncek, F. Reduction of rise in blood pressure and cortisol release during stress by ginkgo biloba extract (EGB 761) in healthy volunteers. *J Physiol Pharmacol.* Sep 2002;53(3):337-48.

Jia-Shi, Z., Halpern, G.M., Jones, K. The scientific rediscovery of a precious ancient Chinese herbal regimen: cordyceps sinensis—part I. *The J of Alternative and Complementary Medicine.* 1998;4(3):289-303.

Jia-Shi, Z., Halpern, G.M., Jones, K. The scientific rediscovery of a precious ancient Chinese herbal regimen: cordyceps sinensis—part II. *The Journal of Alternative and Complementary Medicine.* 1998;4(4):429-57.

Johnson, T.E. Recent results: biomarkers of aging. *Exp. Gerontol.* 2006;41:1243-6.

Julius, S. Effect of sympathetic overactivity on cardiovascular prognosis in hypertension. *Eur Heart J.* 1998;19 Suppl F:F14-8.

Keller, U. From obesity to diabetes. *Int J Vitam Nutr Res.* Jul 2006;76(4):172-7.

Kelly, G.S. Nutritional and botanical interventions to assist with the adaptation to stress. *Altern Med Rev.* Aug 1999;4(4):249-65.

Kelly, G. Clinical applications of N-acetylcysteine. *Alt Med Rev.* 1998;3(2):114-27.

Kelly, J.J., Mangos, G., Williamson, P.M., Whitworth, J.A. Cortisol and hypertension. *Clin Exp Pharmacol Physiol.* 1998;25 Suppl:S51-56.

Kelly, J.J., Tam, S.H., Williamson, P.M., Lawson, J., Whitworth, J.A. The nitric oxide system and cortisol-induced hypertension in humans. *Clin Exp Pharmacol Physiol.* 1998;25:945-6.

Keltikangas-J'arvinen, L., R'aikk'onen, K., Hautanen, A. Type A behavior and vital exhaustion as related to the metabolic hormonal variables of the hypothalamic-pituitary-adrenal axis. *Behav Med.* Spring 1996; 22:15-22.

Kemnitz, J.W., Roecker, E.B., Weindruch, R., Elson, D.F., Baum, S.T., Bergman, R.N. Dietary restriction increases insulin sensitivity and lowers blood glucose in rhesus monkeys. *Am J Physiol.* 1994;266:E540-E547.

Kempuraj, D., Madhappan, B. Flavonols inhibit proinflammatory mediator release, intracellular calcium ion levels and protein kinase C theta phosphorylation in human mast cells. *Br J Pharmacol.* Aug 2005;145(7):933-44.

Kendler, B.S. Taurine: an overview of its role in preventive medicine. *Prev Med.* 1989;18(1):79-100.

Khani, S., Tayek, J.A. Cortisol increases gluconeogenesis in humans: its role in the metabolic syndrome. *Clin Sci (Long).* Dec 2001;101(6):739-47.

Kim, M.J., Aiken, J.M., Havighurst, T., Hollander, J., Ripple, M.O., Weindruch, R. Adult-onset energy restriction of rhesus monkeys attenuates oxidative stress-induced cytokine expression by peripheral blood mononuclear cells. *J. Nutr.* 1997;127:2293-301.

Kloting, N., Bluher, M. Extended longevity and insulin signaling in adipose tissue. *Exp Gerontol.* 2005;40:878-83.

Knoops, K. Mediterranean diet, lifestyle factors, and 10-year mortality in elderly European men and women. *JAMA.* 2004;292:1433-9.

Kodama, M., Kodama, T. Vitamin C infusion treatment enhances cortisol production of the adrenal via the pituitary ACTH route. *In Vivo.* Nov-Dec 1994;8(6):1079-85.

Krahenbuhl, S., Hasler, F. Kinetics and dynamics of orally administered 18 beta-glycyrrhetinic acid in humans. *J Clin Endocrinol Metab.* Mar 1994;78(3):581-5.

Kremer, J.M. N-3 fatty acid supplements in rheumatoid arthritis. *Am J Clin Nutr.* 2000;71 Suppl:S349-51.

Kuo, Y.C., Tsai, W.G. Cordyceps sinesis as an immunomodulatory agent. *Am J Chin Med.* 1996;24(2):111-25.

Laferrere, B., Abraham, C. Inhibiting endogenous cortisol blunts the meal-entrained rise in serum leptin. *J Clin Endocrinol Metab.* Jun 2006;91(6):2232-8.

Lane, J.D., Pieper, C.F. Caffeine affects cardiovascular and neuroendocrine activation at work and home. *Psychosom Med.* Jul-Aug 2002;64(4):595-603.

Lanfranco, F., Giordana, R., Pellegrino, M., Gianotti, L., Ramunni, J., Picu, A., et al. Free fatty acids exert an inhibitory effect on adrenocorticotropin and cortisol secretion in humans. *J Clin Endocrinol Metab.* Mar 2004;89(3):1385-90.

Larre, C., Rochat de la Vallee, E. Rooted in spirit: the heart of Chinese medicine. Barrytown, NY: Station Hill Press; 1995.

Larson-Meyer, D.E., Heilbronn, L.K., Redman, L.M. Effect of calorie restriction with or without exercise on insulin sensitivity, beta-cell function, fat cell size and ectopic lipid in overweight subjects. *Diabetes Care.* 2006;29:1337-44.

Larsson, B., Seidell, J., Svardsudd, K.,Welir, L. Tibblin, G., Wilhelmesen, L., et al. Obesity, adipose tissue distribution and health in men—the study of men born in 1913. *Appetite.* 1989;13:37-44.

Laughter—can it keep you healthy? *Mayo Clinic Health Letter.* March 1993, p6.

Lee, J.H., O'Keefe, J.H., Bell, D., Hensrud, D.D., Holick, M.F. Vitamin D deficiency an important, common, and easily treatable cardiovascular risk factor? *J Am Coll Cardiol.* May 26 2009;53(21):2011-3.

Lee, K.M., Yeo, M. Protective mechanism of epigallocatechin-3-gallate against Helicobacter pylori-induced gastric epithelial cytotoxicity via the blockage of TLR-4 signaling. *Helicobacter.* Dec 2004;9(6):632-42.

Le Gal, C., Cathebras P., Struby K. Pharmeton capsules in the treatment of functional fatigue: a double blind study versus placebo evaluated by a new methodology. *Phytother Res* 1996; 10;49-53

Leu, S.F., Chien, C.H., Tseng, C.Y., Kuo, Y.M., Huang, B.M. The in vivo effect of cordyceps sinensis mycelium on plasma corticosterone level in male mouse. *Biol Pharm Bull.* Sep 2005;28(9):1722-5.

Lewis, J.G., Nakajin, S. Circulating levels of isoflavones and markers of 5alpha-reductase activity are higher in Japanese compared with New Zealand males: what is the role of circulating steroids in prostate disease? *Steroids.* Dec 15 2005;70(14):974-9.

Lombard, C.B. What is the role of food in preventing depression and improving mood, performance and cognitive function? *Med J Aust.* 2000;173 Suppl:S104-5.

Lovallo, W.R., al'Absi, M., Blick, K., Whitsett, T.L., Wilson, M.F. Stress-like adrenocorticotropin responses to caffeine in young healthy men. *Pharmacol Biochem Behav.* Nov 1996;55(3):365-9.

Lovallo W.R., Whitsett T.L. Caffeine stimulation of cortisol secretion across the waking hours in relation to caffeine intake levels. *Psychosom Med.* Sep-Oct 2005;67(5):734-9.

Lu, H.C. (trans). The Yellow Emperor's Classic of Internal Medicine and the Difficult Classic. Vancouver, B.C.: Academy of Oriental Heritage; 1978.

Ludwig ,D. The glycemic index. *JAMA.* May 3 2002;287(18):2414-23.

Ludwig, D.S., Majzoub, J.A., Al-Zahrani, A., Dallal, G.E., Blanco, I., Roberts, S.B. High glycemic index foods, overeating, and obesity. *Pediatrics.* 1999;103(3):E26.

Ludwig, H., Spiteller, M., Egger, H.J. Correlation of emotional stress and physical exertions with urinary metabolite profiles. *J Isr Chem.* 1997;16:7-11.

MacIntosh, A., Ball, K. The effects of a short program of detoxification in disease-free individuals. *Altern Ther Health Med,* 2000;6(4):70-6.

Maksymowych, A.B., Daniel, V., Litwack, G. Pyridoxal phosphate as a regulator of the glucocorticoid receptor. *Ann N Y Acad Sci.* 1990;585:438-51.

Mandel, S.A., Avramovich-Tirosh, Y., Reznichenko, L., Zheng, H., Weinreb, O., Amit, T., et al. Multifunctional activities of green tea catechins in neuroportection. Modulation of cell survival genes, iron-dependent oxidative stress and PKC signaling pathway. *Neuro-signals.* 2005;14(1-2);46-60.

Manolagas, S.C., Provvedini, D.M., Tsoukas, C.D. Interactions of 1,25-dihydroxyvitamin D3 and the immune system. *Mol Cell Endocrinol.* 1985;43:113-22.

Markus,R., Panhuysen, G., Tuiten, A., Koppeschaar, H. Effects of food on cortisol and mood in vulnerable subjects under controllable and uncontrollable stress. *Physiol Behav* 2000 Aug-Sep:70 (3-4) 333-42.

Mao, T.J., van de Water, J. Modulation of TNF-alpha secretion in peripheral blood mononuclear cells by cocoa flavanols and procyanidins. *Dev Immunol.* Sep 2002;9(3):135-41.

Mattsson, C., Reynolds, R.M. Combined receptor antagonist stimulation of the hypothalamic-pituitary-adrenal axis test identifies impaired negative feedback sensitivity to cortisol in obese men. *J Clin Endocrinol Metab.* Apr 2009;94(4):1347-52.

Mayer, G., Kroger, M., Meier-Ewert, K. Effects of vitamin B12 on performance and circadian rhythm in normal subjects. *Neuropsychopharmacology.* Nov 1996;15(5):456-64.

McEwen, B.S. Protective and damaging effects of stress mediators. *N Engl J Med.* 1998;338:171-9.

McEwen, B.S. Stress, adaptation, and disease: allostasis and allostatic load. *Annals New York Academy of Sciences.* May 1;1998; 840:33-44.

McEwen, B.S., Wingfield, J.C. The concept of allostasis in biology and biomedicine. *Horm Behav.* Jan 2003;43(1):2-15.

McEwen, B.S. The neurobiology of stress: from serendipity to clinical relevance. *Brain Res.* Dec 15 2000;886(1-2):172-189.

Merton, T. The way of Chuang Tzu. Boston, Shambala Press 1992.

Michalsen, A., Schneider, S., Rodenbeck, A., Ludtke, R., Huether, G., Dobos, G.J. The short-term effects of fasting on the neuroendocrine system in patients with chronic pain syndromes. *Nutr Neurosci.* Feb 2003;6(1):11-8.

Milagro, F.I., Campion, J., Martinez, J.A. 11-beta Hydroxysteroid dehydrogenase type 2 expression in white adipose tissue is strongly correlated with adiposity. *J of Steroid Biochemistry and Molecular Biology.* Apr 2007;104(1-2):81-4.

Mind/body medicine: how to use your mind for better health. Goleman, D., Gurin, J., Eds. New York: Consumer Reports Books; 1993, p.80.

Mischoulon, D., Fava, M. Docosahexanoic acid and omega-3 fatty acids in depression. *Psychiatr Clin North Am.* 2000;23(4):785-94.

Mochizuki, M., Hasegawa, N. Therapeutic efficacy of pycnogenol in experimental inflammatory bowel diseases. *Phytother Res.* Dec 2004;18(12):1027-8.

Monroe, J., Brostoff,J., Food allergy and migraine *Lancet* July 5,1980

Monteleone, P. Effects of phosphatidylserine on the neuroendocrine response to physical stress in humans. *Neuroendocrinology.* Sep 1990;52(3):243-8.

Monteleone, P. Blunting by chronic phosphatidylserine administration of the stress-induced activation of the hypothalamo-pituitary-adrenal axis in health men. *Eur J Clin Pharmacol.* 1992;(41):385-8.

Moro, J.R., Iwata, M., Von Andriano, U.H. Vitamin effects on the immune system: vitamins A and D take center stage. *Nat Rev Immunol.* Sep 2008;8(9):685-98.

Muhtz, C., Zyriax, B.C. Depressive symptoms and metabolic risk: effects of cortisol and gender. *Psychoneuroendocrinology.* Aug 2009;34(7):1004-11.

Muller, J.E., Tofler, G.H., Willich, S.N., Stone, P.H. Circadian variation of cardiovascular disease and sympathetic activity. *J Cardiovasc Pharmacol.* 1987;10 Suppl 2:S104-9.

Munger, K.L., Zhang, S.M., O'Reilly, E. Vitamin D intake and the incidence of multiple sclerosis. *Neurology.* 2004;62:60-5.

Murck, J., Song, C. Ethyl-Eicosapentaenoate and dexamethasone resistence in therapy-refractory depression. *Int J Neurophyshopharmacol.* Sep 2004;7(3):341-9.

Nanda, R. Food intolerance and the irritable bowel syndrome. *Gut.* 1989;30:1099-104.

National Institute of Mental Health. Facts about anxiety disorders. http://www.nimh.nih.gov/anxiety; January 1999.

Nestel, P.J. Fish oil and cardiovascular disease: lipids and arterial function. *Am J Clin Nutr.* 2000;71 Suppl:S228-31.

Nuttall, F.Q., Gannon, M.D. The metabolic response to a high-protein, low-carbohydrate diet in men with type 2 diabetes mellitus. *Metabolism.* Feb 2006;55(2):243-51.

O'Keefe, J.H., Gheewala, N.M., O'Keefe, J.O. Dietary strategies for improving post-prandial glucose, lipids, inflammation, and cardiovascular health. *J Am Coll Cardiol.* 2008;51:249-55.

Ornish, D. Love and survival. New York: Harper Collins; 1997.

Packer, L., Witt, E.H., Tritschler, H.J. Alpha-lipoic acid as a biological antioxidant. *Free Rad Biol Med.* 1995;19(2):227-50.

Palomer, X., Gonzalez-Clemente, J.M., Blanco-Vaca, F., Mauricio, D. Role of vitamin D in the pathogenesis of type 2 diabetes mellitus. *Diabetes Obes Metab.* Mar 2008;10(3):185-97.

Panossian, A., Wikman, G., Wagner, H. Plant adaptogens. III. Earlier and more recent aspects and concepts on their mode of action. *Phytomedicine.* Oct 1999;6(4):287-300.

Parillo, M., Rivellese, A.A., Ciardullo, A.V. A high monounsaturated-fat/low-carbohydrate diet improves peripheral insulin sensitivity in non-insulin dependent diabetic patients. *Metabolism.* 1992;41:1373-8.

Pattison, D.J., Symmons, D.P. Dietary beta-cryptoxanthin and inflammatory polyarthritis: results from a population-based prospective study. *Am J Clin Nutr.* Aug 2005;82(2):451-5.

Paulose, C.S., Dakshinamurti, K., Packer, S., Stephens, N.L. Sympathetic stimulation and hypertension in the pyridoxine-deficient adult rat. *Hypertension.* 1998;11:387-91.

Pradhan, A.D., Manson, J.A.E., Rifai, N., Buring, J.E., Ridker, P.M. C-reactive protein, interleukin 6, and risk of developing type 2 diabetes mellitus. *JAMA.* 2001;286:327-34.

Prasad, K. Hypocholesterolemic and antiatherosclerotic effect of flax lignan complex isolated from flaxseed. *Atherosclerosis.* Apr 2005;179(2):269-75.

Reaven, G. Metabolic syndrome. *Circulation.* Jul 16 2002;106:286-8.

Resnick, L.M. Ionic basis of hypertension, insulin resistance, vascular disease, and related disorders: the mechanism of "syndrome X." *Am J Hypertens.* 1993;6:123S-134S.

Reynolds, R.M., Godfrey, K.M. Stress responsiveness in adult life: influence of mother's diet in late pregnancy. *J Clin Endocrinol Metab.* Mar 6 2007;92(6):2208-10.

Rideout, C.A., Linden, W., Barr, S.I. High cognitive dietary restraint is associated with increased cortisol excetion in postmenopausal women. *J Gerontol A Biol Sci Med Sci.* Jun 2006;61(6):628-33.

Rigden, S., Barrager, E., Bland, J. Evaluation of the effect of a modified entero-hepatic resuscitation program in chronic fatigue syndrome patients. *J Adv Med.* 1998;11(4):247-62.

Rimm, E.B., Willett, W.C. Folate and vitamin B6 from diet and supplements in relation to risk of coronary heart disease among women. *JAMA.* 1998;279:359-64.

Riordan, A.M. Treatment of active Crohn's disease by exclusion diet: East Anglian Multicenter control trial. *Lancet.* 1990;335:816-9.

Rivellese, A., Riccardi, G., Giacco, A. Effect of dietary fibre on glucose control and serum lipoproteins in diabetic patients. *Lancet.* 1980;2:447-50.

Robinson, K., Arheart, K., Refsum, H. Low circulating folate and vitamin B6 concentrations: risk factors for stroke, peripheral vascular disease, and coronary artery disease. European COMAC Group. *Circulation.* 1998;97:437-43.

Rosenman, R.H. Results of the multicenter antihypertensive treatment trials. Therapeutic implications and the role of the sympathetic nervous system. *Am J Hypertens.* 1989;2:313S-338S.

Rosmond, R., Bjorntorp, P. Alterations in the hypothalamic-pituitary-adrenal axis in metabolic syndrome. *The Endocrinologist.* 2001;11:491-7.

Rosmond, R., Holm, G., Bjorntorp, P. Food-induced cortisol secretion in relation to anthropometric, metabolic and hemodynamic variables in men. *Int. J. Obes.* Apr 2000 24:416-22.

Roubenoff, R., Castaneda, C. Sarcopenia—understanding the dynamics of aging muscle. *JAMA.* 2001;286(10):230-1.

Rowland, I., Faughnam, M. Bioavailability of phyto-estrogens. *Br J Nutr.* Jun 2003;89 Suppl 1:S45-58.

Ruhe, R.C., McDonald, R.B. Use of antioxidant nutrients in the prevention and treatment of type 2 diabetes. *J Am Coll Nutrition.* 2001;20:363S-369S.

Rushmore, T.H., Kong, A. Pharmacogenomics, regulation and signaling pathways of phase I and II drug metabolizing enzymes. *Curr Drug Metab.* Oct 2002;3(5):481-90.

Sabatino, R., Masoro, E.J., McMahan, C.A., Kuhn, R.W. Assessment of the role of the glucocorticoid system in aging processes and in the action of food restriction. *J Gerontol.* 1991;46:B171-B179.

Salmeron, J., Manson, J.E., Stampfer, M.J., Colditz, G.A., Wing, A.L., Willett, W.C. Dietary fiber, glycemic load and risk of non-insulin-dependent diabetes mellitus in women. *JAMA.* 1997;277:472-7.

Salmeron, J., Manson, J.E., Stampfer, M.J., Colditz, G.A., Wing, A.L., Willett, W.C. Dietary fiber, glycemic load and risk of non-insulin-dependent diabetes mellitus in men. *Diabetes Care.* 1997;20(4):545-50.

Sapolsky, R., Krey, L., McEwen, B. The neuroendocrinology of stress and aging: the glucocorticoid cascade hypothesis. *Endocrinol.* 1986;Rev.7:284-301.

Schinner, S. Adipocyte-derived products induce the transcription of the StAR promoter and stimulate aldosterone and cortisol secretion from adrenocortical cells through the Wnt-signaling pathway. *Int J Obes (Lond.).* Jan 9 2007;31:864-70.

Seeman, T.E., Singer, B.H., Rowe, J.W., Horwitz, R.I., McEwen, B.S. The price of adaptation—allostatic load and its health consequences: MacArthur studies of successful aging. *Arch. Intern. Med.* 1997;157:2259-68.

Shibata, S. A drug over the millennia: pharmacognosy, chemistry, and pharmacology of licorice. *Journal of the Pharmaceutical Society of Japan.* Oct 2000;120(10):849-62.

Siguel, E.N., Schaefer, E.J. Aging & nutritional requirements of EFAs. In: Beare, J., ed. *Dietary Fats*, AO CS, 1989.

Siguel, E.N. Cancerostatic effect of vegetable diets. *Nut and Cancer.* 1983;4:285-9.

Siguel, E.N., Lerman R.H. Trans fatty acid metabolism in patients with angiographically documented coronary artery disease. *Am J Cardiol.* 1993;71(11):916-20.

Siguel, E. The role of essential fatty acids in health and disease. Nutrition Issue. *Contemporary Therapy.* 1994;20(9):500-10.

Simopoulos, A.P., Salem, N. Jr. N-3 fatty acids in eggs from range-fed Greek chickens. *N Engl J Med.* 1989;32(20):1412.

Sinclair, H.M. Essential fatty acids—an historical perspective. *Biochem Soc Trans.* 1990;18:756-61.

Singh, R.B., Pella, D. Can brain dysfunction be a predisposing factor for metabolic syndrome? *Biomed Pharmacother.* Oct 2004;58 Suppl 1:S56-68.

Skantze, H.B., Kaplan, J., Pettersson, K., Manuck, S., Blomqvist, N., Kyes, R., et al. Psychosocial stress causes endothelial injury in cynomolgus monkeys via beta 1-adrenoceptor activation. *Atherosclerosis.* 1998;136:153-61.

Smith, A. Stress, breakfast cereal consumption and cortisol. *Nutritional Neuroscience.* April 2002;5(2):141-4.

Sohal, R.S., Mockett, R.J., Orr, W.C. Mechanisms of aging: an appraisal of the oxidative stress hypothesis. *Free Radic Biol Med.* 2002;33:575-86.

Sohal, R.S., Weindruch, R. Oxidative stress, caloric restriction and aging. *Science* 1996;273:59-63.

Spence, J.D., Thornton, T. The effect of flax seed cultivars with differing content of alpha-oinolenic acid and lignans on responses to mental stress. *J Am Coll Nutr.* Dec 2003;22(6):494-501.

Sreejayan Rao, M.N. Nitric oxide scavenging by curcuminoids. *J. Pharm Pharmocol* 1997:49:105-7.

Starks, M.A., Starks, S.L., Kingsley, M., Purpura, M., Jäger, R. The effects of phosphatidylserine on endocrine response to moderate intensity exercise. *J of the International Society of Sports Nutrition.* Jul 2008;5:11.

Steptoe, A., Gibson, E.L., Vuononvirta, R., Williams, E.D., Hamer, M., Rycroft, J.A. The effects of tea on psychophysiological stress responsivity and post-stress recovery: a randomized double-blind trial. *Psychopharmacology (Berl).* Jan 2007;190(1):81-9.

Steptoe, A., Kunz-Ebrecht, S.R. Central adiposity and cortisol responses to waking in middle-aged men and women. *Int J Obes Relat Metab Disord.* Sep 2004;28(9):1168-73.

Straus, D.S. Nutritional regulation of hormones and growth factors that control mammalian growth. *FASEB J.* 1994;8:6-12.

Swaab, D.F., Bao, A.M. The stress system in the human brain in depression and neurodegeneration. *Ageing Res Rev.* May 2005;4(2):131-94.

Tahiliani, A.G., Beinlich, C.J. Pantothenic acid in health and disease. *Vitam Horm.* 1991;46:165-228.

Tauchmanova, L., Rossi, R., Biondi, B., Pulcrano, M., Nuzzo, V. Palmieri, E.A. Patients with subclinical Cushing's syndrome due to adrenal adenoma have increased cardiovascular risk. *J Clin Endocrinol Metab.* Nov 2002;87(11):4869-71.

Teitelbaum, J. Effective treatment of chronic fatigue syndrome and fibromyalgia: a randomized, double blind, placebo-controlled, intent-to-treat study. *J Chronic Fatigue Syndrome.* 2001;8:3-28.

Thompson, L.U., Chen, J.M., et al. Dietary flaxseed alters tumor biological markers in postmenopausal breast cancer. *Clin Cancer Res.* May 15 2005;11(10):3828-35.

Trichopoulou, A. Modified Mediterranean diet and survival epic—elderly perspective cohort study. *British Medical Journal.* Apr 30 2005;330:799-805.

Tuck, M., Corry, D. More on adrenal activity in the metabolic syndrome. *Curr Hypertens Rep.* Apr 2002;4(2):103-4.

Tully, D.B., Allgood, V.E., Cidlowski, J.A. Modulation of steroid receptor-mediated gene expression by vitamin B6. *FASEB J.* 1994;8:343-9.

Uusitupa, M., Schwab, U., Makimattila, S. Effects of two high-fat diets with different fatty acid compositions on glucose and lipid metabolism in healthy young women. *Am J Clin Nutr.* 1994;59:1310-6.

Van Cauter, E., Spiegel K. Metabolic consequences of sleep and sleep loss. *Sleep Med.* Sep 2008;9 Suppl 1:S23-8.

Van Herpen-Broekmans, W.M., Klopping-Ketelaars, I.A., Serum carotenoids and vitamins in relation to markers of endothelial function and inflammation. *Eur J Epidemiol.* 2004;19(10):915-21.

Veith, I. Huang Ti Nei Ching Su Wen: the Yellow Emperor's Classic of Internal Medicine. Berkeley, CA: University of California Press; 1949.

Vessby, B., Unsitupa, M., Hermansen, K. Substituting dietary saturated for monounsaturated fat impairs insulin sensitivity in healthy men and women: the KANWU study. *Diabetologia.* 2001;44:312-9.

Vicennati ,V. Response of the hypothalamic pituitary adrenocortical axis to high protein and high carbohydrate meals. *J of Clin Endocrinology and Metabolism.* 2002;87(8):3984-8.

Villardita, C. Multicentre clinical trial of brain phosphatidylserine in elderly patients with intellectual deterioration. *Clin Trials J.* 1987;(24):84-93.

Villareal, D.T., Apovian, C.M., Kushner, R.F., Clein, S; American Society for Nutrition; NAASO, The Obesity Society. Obesity in older adults: technical review and position statement of the American Society for Nutrition and NAASO, The Obesity Society. *Am J Clin Nutr.* 2005;82:923-34.

Villareal, D.T., Fontana, L., Weiss, E.P. Bone mineral density response to caloric restriction-induced weight loss or exercise-induced weight loss: a randomized controlled trial. *Arch Intern Med.* 2006;166:2502-10.

Vina, J., Perez, C., Furukawa, T. Effect of oral glutathione on hepatic glutathione levels in rats and mice. *Br J Nutr.* 1989;62(3):683-91.

Vogelzangs, N., Beekman, A.T., Dik, M.G., Bremmer, M.A., Comijs, H.C., Hoogendijk, W.J., et al. Late-life depression, cortisol, and the metabolic syndrome. *Am J Geriatr Psychiatry*. Aug 2009;17(8):716-21.

Vogelzangs, N., Suthers, K. Hypercortisolemic depression is associated with the metabolic syndrome in late-life. *Pschoneuroendocrinology*. Feb 2007;32(2):151-9.

Volek, J., Sharman, M., Love, D., Avery, N., Gomez, A., Scheett, T., et al. Body composition and hormonal responses to a carbohydrate-restricted diet. *Metabolism*. Jul 2002;51(7):864-70.

Waldschlager, J., Bergemann, C. Flax-seed extracts with phytoestrogenic effects on a hormone receptor-positive tumour cell line. *Anticancer Res*. May-Jun 2005;(3A):1817-22.

Walford, R.L., Mock, D., Verdery, R., MacCallum, T. Calorie restriction in biosphere 2: alterations in physiologic, hematologic, hormonal, and biochemical parameters in humans restricted for a 2-year period. *J Gerontol A Biol Sci Med Sci*. 2002;57:B211-B224.

Walker, B.R. Cortisol—cause and cure for metabolic syndrome? *Diabet Med*. Dec 2006;23(12):1281-8.

Walker, B.R. Steroid metabolism in metabolic syndrome X. *Best Pract Res Clin Endocrinol Metab*. Mar 2001;15(1):111-22.

Walker, B.R., Andrew, R. Tissue production of cortisol by 11beta-hydroxysteroid dehydrogenase type 1 and metabolic disease. *Ann NY Acad Sci*. Nov 2006;1083:165-84.

Wang, S., Chen, S. Genistein protects dopaminergic neurons by inhibiting microglial activation. *Neuroreport*. Feb 28 2005;16(3):267-70.

Watkins, B.A., Li, Y., Lippman, H.E. Omega-3 polyunsaturated fatty acids and skeletal health. *Exp Biol Med*. 2001;226(6):485-97.

Weber, M.A. Sympathetic nervous system and hypertension. Therapeutic perspectives. *Am J Hypertens*. 1989;2:147S-152S.

Weber-Hamann, B., Hentschel, F., Kniest, A., Deuschle, M., Colla, M., Lederbogen, F., et al. Hypercortisolemic depression is associated with increased intra-abdominal fat. *Psychosom Med.* Mar-Apr 2002;64(2):274-7.

Weindruck, R., Walford, R.L. The Retardation of Aging and Disease by Dietary Restriction. Springfield, IL: Charles C. Thomas Publisher; 1988.

Weiss, E.P., Racette, S.B., Villareal, D.T. Improvements in glucose tolerance and insulin action induced by increasing energy expenditure or decreasing energy intake: a randomized controlled trial. *Am J Clin Nutr.* 2006;84:1033-42.

Williams, J.K., Kaplan, J.R., Manuck, S.B. Effects of psychosocial stress on endothelium-mediated dilation of atherosclerotic arteries in cynomolgus monkeys. *J Clin Invests.* 1993;92:1819-23.

Williams, S.N., Shih, H., Guenette, D.K. Comparative studies on the effects of green tea extracts and individual tea catechins on human CYP1A gene expression. *Chem Biol Interact.* 2000;128(3):211-29.

Wood, R., Kubena, K., O'Breien, B., Tseng, S., Martin, G. Effect of butter, mono- and poly-unsaturated fatty acid-enriched butter, trans fatty acid margarine, and zero trans fatty acid margarine on serum lipids and lipoproteins in healthy men. *J Lipid Res.* Jan 1993;34(1):1-11.

Worsley, J.R. Classical Five-Element acupuncture: the five elements and the officials, Vol. III. J.R. & J.B. Worsley, Publishers; 1998.

Yehuda, S., Rabinovitz, S., Mostofsky, D.I. Mixture of essential fatty acids lowers test anxiety. *Nutr Neurosci.* Aug 2005;8(4):265-7.

Yehuda, S., Rabinovitz, S. Fatty acid mixture counters stress changes in cortisol, cholesterol, and impair learning. *Int J Neurosci.* 2000;101(1-4):73-87.

Zadshir, A., Tareen, N., Pan, D., Norris, K., Martins, D. The prevalence of hypovitaminosis D among US adults: data from the NHANES III. *Ethn Dis.* 2005;15(4 Suppl 5):S5-97-101.

Zhu, J.S., Halpern, G.M., Jones, K. The scientific rediscovery of a precious ancient Chinese herbal medicine: cordyceps sinesis: part I. *J Altern Complement Med* 1998;4(3):289-303

Zitterman, A., Frisch, S., Berthold, H.K., Gotting, C., Kuhn, J., Kleesiek, K., et al. Vitamin D supplementation enhances the beneficial effects of weight loss on cardiovascular disease risk markers. *Am J Clin Nutr.* May 2009;89(5):1321-7.

Zittermann, A. Vitamin D in preventive medicine: are we ignoring the evidence? *Br J Nutr.* 2003;89:552-72.

Index

Page numbers in *italics* refer to tables

Manufactured By: RR Donnelley
Breinigsville, PA USA
May, 2010